Wolfgang Fürweger

Care atlases for managing regional healthcare systems

Wolfgang Fürweger

Care atlases for managing regional healthcare systems

Opportunities and challenges - the example of the federal state of Salzburg

ScienciaScripts

Imprint

Cover image: www.ingimage.com

This book is a translation from the original published under ISBN 978-620-0-44951-1.

Publisher:
Sciencia Scripts
is a trademark of
Dodo Books Indian Ocean Ltd. and OmniScriptum S.R.L publishing group

120 High Road, East Finchley, London, N2 9ED, United Kingdom
Str. Armeneasca 28/1, office 1, Chisinau MD-2012, Republic of Moldova, Europe
Printed at: see last page
ISBN: 978-620-3-98436-1

Contents

Abstract

Demographic change is forcing healthcare systems at all levels to reorganise their care structures. In Salzburg, the idea was born to develop a regional, cross-sectoral care atlas as an information and planning tool for politicians, administrators, experts and the population. This book summarises the basis for this: It uses the literature and three best-practice examples from the USA and Germany to illustrate what geographical representations in health reporting can and cannot achieve and develops a checklist for a good health care atlas. In interviews with experts, the opportunities, requirements and challenges for a regional, cross-sectoral health care atlas for the federal state of Salzburg are analysed. The interviews show that a regional project for Salzburg should be started as an interactive online platform on a small scale and continuously developed during operation.

CHAPTER 1

1 Introduction

1.1 Demographic change as a challenge

Demographic change is currently the biggest challenge facing healthcare systems in western industrialised countries. This realisation is by no means new: as early as 2010, Da-Cruz and Hermann in Germany, for example, pointed out: "Demographic changes are becoming a stress test for the healthcare system. Morbidity is increasing considerably and a significant increase in the prevalence of many diseases is forecast. These developments present service providers with particular challenges that are already the subject of heated debate." (Da Cruz/Hermann, 2010, p. 623)
At this time in Austria, the first representatives of the baby boomer generation, i.e. those born between 1946 and 1964, were able to retire regularly after thousands of early retirements per year and the population pyramid began to tilt (Furweger, 2023). Since 2010, this trend has gained further momentum and will continue: in 2018, the proportion of 80-year-olds and older in Austria was 5 per cent of the population, by 2030 it is expected to rise to 6.7 per cent and by 2050 to 11.2 per cent. In absolute figures, this means that in 2018 there were 438,000 people aged 80 and over living in Austria; according to projections, this figure will rise to 621,000 in 2030 and 1.07 million in 2050. (Statistics Austria, 2019)
This development naturally affects all areas of society, but in particular medical and nursing care, as the population is not only getting older, but also potentially sicker and more in need of care: "In the healthcare sector in particular, the demand for medical care is increasing as society ages ... However, this considerable increase in demand is offset by comparatively unfavourable physician demographics." (Famira-Muhlberger/Streicher, 2020). This study, commissioned by the Austrian Institute of Economic Research (WIFO), focussed specifically on medical care. However, in the author's opinion, this finding also applies to intramural and extramural care.
The retirement of employees from the baby boomer generation from the healthcare system is not in itself a cause for concern. However, the rising number of retirements is being accompanied by falling birth rates. Recent figures are available for the federal state of Salzburg - they show the effects of this development particularly clearly: 526,700 people lived in the state in 2010. 65,300 (12.4 per cent) belonged to the age cohort of 15 to 25-year-olds, i.e. were potential career starters. In 2022, the total population was already 562,600 people due to domestic immigration and immigration from other countries, an increase of 6.8 per cent compared to 2010. At the same time, the number of 15 to 25-year-olds fell by 6,100 to 59,200 in the same

period. Within the cohorts, this meant a decline of 15.3 per cent. In relation to the total population, the number of potential career entrants fell from 12.4 to 10.5 per cent in just twelve years. By 2032, the total population in the federal state of Salzburg is expected to grow to 577,000 people due to immigration. At the same time, the number of 15 to 25-year-olds will continue to fall - to 54,000 people or 9.4 per cent of the total population. (Furweger, 2023) That means: In Austria, there are more and more old and elderly people and fewer and fewer young and younger people who could potentially work in the healthcare system. The staff shortage in the healthcare system will therefore continue to increase.

1.2 A regional supply atlas as a tool for needs-based planning

From diagnosis to possible therapies, which the author believes are necessary: On the one hand, employers in the healthcare system must endeavour to recruit as many young people as possible - while naturally competing with other sectors. Existing employees must be kept in the system for as long as possible by taking measures to promote their physical and mental health - if possible beyond the statutory retirement age. And the trend towards part-time work should be stopped, for example by offering more and better childcare or making full-time work more financially attractive. These aspects were interesting topics for our own work, but can only be touched on here for reasons of space.

In addition, the healthcare system as a whole must become more needs-orientated. Because in the not-so-distant future, fewer young and younger people will have to provide medical treatment and care to more old and elderly people. Digitalisation provides important tools for this, such as surgical robots or digital patient charts. However, the use of technology and personnel must also be more targeted. On the one hand, this can be achieved by streamlining and reorganising existing processes; on the other hand, it also requires needs-based planning of care structures - a particular challenge in the Austrian healthcare system.

The central elements of regional healthcare policy and care planning are the Austrian Health Structure Plan (OSG) and the respective Regional Health Structure Plans (RSG) of the federal states (e.g. Land Salzburg 2019; EPIG 2019). These are each created for five years on the basis of data collected retrospectively. There are also separate structural plans for the inpatient and outpatient sectors. In the domestic healthcare system, the path to the future is therefore currently being planned by looking in two rear-view mirrors, each pointing in a different direction. This is where an idea comes in that was developed in the federal state of Salzburg at the

Research and Innovation Centre for Public Health and Health Care Research at Paracelsus Medical University (PMU) and taken up by stakeholders from Salzburg University Hospital and the health department of the state of Salzburg: a cross-sectoral health care atlas for the federal state of Salzburg as a presentation and planning tool for regional health care administration and policy.

The author has taken up this idea and made it the subject of his master's thesis. The specific aim of this thesis is to present the basis for a regional, cross-sector atlas of health care in Austria. The central research question is therefore: How should a regional, cross-sector atlas of healthcare provision be structured for an Austrian federal state and what opportunities and challenges arise from its implementation? As the author is the spokesperson for the Salzburg regional clinics and these are the largest healthcare provider in the federal state of Salzburg, the basis for a regional, cross-sector atlas of healthcare provision is developed using the example of the Austrian federal state of Salzburg. It could be argued that a cross-sector atlas of healthcare provision should not be limited to one region, but should be approached on a national level. However, the political reality in Austria stands in the way of this: The domestic healthcare system is not only characterised by shared responsibilities and very complex financial flows, but also has a highly decentralised structure. Basically, there are ten healthcare systems in a country that is almost 84,000 square kilometres in size and has 9.1 million inhabitants: the federal system and one for each of the nine federal states. The author therefore sees a regional care atlas as a pragmatic and sensible solution. The wheel does not have to be completely reinvented. Atlases are not a recent invention in the research of medical care and have become increasingly popular in health services research in recent years: "Interest in the cartographic representation of medical care topics has increased significantly in recent years. This can be seen in the large number of health atlases that have been published internationally in the recent past." (Mangiapane, 2014).

1.3 Structure and organisation of the work

The aim of this master's thesis is to present the principles, requirements/desires, opportunities and challenges for a regional, cross-sector atlas of healthcare provision. The actual implementation in the federal state of Salzburg would be the subject of a further project, which would require appropriate financial and human resources. Ulrich et al. (2017) note that health data is also available for small regions, but that processing and analysing it is time-consuming and expensive.

This paper consists of two parts: In the first part, the difference between epidemiological atlases and health care atlases is presented based on the literature. Subsequently, best-practice examples are used to work out what cartographic representations in general and geo-information systems and atlases in particular can and cannot achieve in health services research. A gap in knowledge also became apparent to the author when studying the literature: When searching for "Health AND Mapping" (cf. Augustin et al., 2018) on PubMed, more than 5,700 articles are displayed for 2023 alone. However, the author has not found a dedicated list of quality criteria for a good healthcare atlas. Such a catalogue of criteria is therefore drawn up in the discussion on the basis of the literature and the author's own considerations. In the second, empirical part, open guideline interviews with experts from the Salzburg health care system are used to ascertain what practical requirements there are for a regional, cross-sectoral health care atlas for an Austrian federal state, what it should or could achieve and what challenges its implementation will entail. The final discussion of the theoretical and empirical part will show that a regional care atlas should be made available digitally and be interactive in accordance with scientific criteria. It should not only be aimed at experts and politicians, but also at a broader, interested public and should not be limited to questions of health services research, but should also consider epidemiological aspects to a limited extent and link the data to projected population development. The literature shows that the geographical representation of both large and small areas can make important contributions to health services research and management. In a study on the influence of the NHS Atlas of Variation in Healthcare on regional NHS decision-makers, Schang et al. (2014) came to the following conclusion: "Our findings illustrate that an Atlas of Variation can support healthcare payers in framing, communicating and prompting the search for strategic problems ..."

1.4 Relevance for practice

A regional, cross-sector atlas of healthcare provision for an Austrian federal state is to be summarised:

- In his presentation, he combines inpatient and outpatient care,
- thereby represent supply structures and processes,
- Integrate health indicators, epidemiology, morbidity and mortality data as far as possible/available,
- take future population trends into account and thus
- Provide a basis for the ongoing management and medium-term planning of regional healthcare policy and provision.

For example, a care atlas was able to show regional overuse or underuse. In conjunction with the forecast of population development, which is available down to municipal level, it was possible to create or relocate health insurance centres in good time, implement telemedical support tools in line with demand or purchase large-scale equipment. The health atlas was also able to address epidemiological issues and show whether certain diseases (e.g. cardiovascular, metabolic, lung diseases, diabetes, juvenile or adult obesity ...) are evenly distributed across the country or whether there are regional focal points. This would allow prevention programmes to be targeted regionally or locally.

With their own regional, cross-sectoral atlases of healthcare provision, Austria's federal states also followed the guideline "Good Practice Health Reporting". The preamble states: "One of its [health monitoring] essential tasks is to interpret data from various data sources. As a health policy control instrument, it provides the empirical basis for rationally justifiable political decisions, it accompanies health policy processes and it offers a basis for participation. At the same time, it is embedded in a political discourse." (Starke et. al., 2019, p. 4). Guideline 4 (subject of the report) states: "Health reporting describes current and data-based defined aspects of the state of health of the population or population groups. It provides descriptions and analyses of health determinants, framework conditions and other health-relevant areas." (Starke et al., 2019, p. 7)

In the author's view, a regional, cross-sectoral health care atlas for an Austrian federal state would be an effective medium for providing the presentations and analyses required in the guideline "Good Practice Health Reporting".

CHAPTER 2

2 Geographical representations in medicine

This chapter begins by defining key terms that are used repeatedly in this work. In addition, the section provides a brief, historical insight into the state of research on geographical representations in medicine and on medical atlases. The differences between epide- miological atlases and health care atlases are presented and the aims of cartographic representations and atlases in health care research are worked out.

2.1 Definitions

For the year 2023, PubMed has more than 6,200 publications with the word "atlas" in the title. Very few of these are atlases in the geographical sense, because as the Dictionary of Geography defines, an atlas is "... a compilation of maps in book form or a series of individual maps that form a factual unit and are intended for common storage (e.g. in a cassette), even if they appear at intervals. It is essential that the cards are harmonised in terms of format, borders, letters, content and graphics. In addition to the printed editions, there are also electronic atlases today, either as atlases for viewing on screen ('view-only atlases') or as interactive multimedia atlases, which allow the linking of map elements with other information, e.g. stored in a database. Numerous atlases are available on the Internet." (Spektrum der Wissenschaft, 2023)

When the term "atlas" is used in this paper, it is to be understood in the sense of this definition. Atlases and maps must be distinguished from *geoinformation systems*, which are also widely used in medicine. Geoinformation systems (GIS) are more than just maps, or rather they extend their utilisation possibilities. They consist of five components: software, hardware,

data, methods and organisation in terms of processes and the provision of resources. (Fletcher-Lartey/Caprarelli, 2016; Thi- Ben et al., 2017). The central visualisation tools are the *layers.* "Data is stored in a GIS on thematic layers, so-called layers, which can be related to each other. Geodata can be divided into vector and raster data. Vector data (or layers) can in turn be differentiated into point, line and polygon layers. Point layers can, for example, include geographical coordinates of facilities such as fast food restaurants, doctors' surgeries or playgrounds, but also regionally occurring events such as criminal offences or cases of illness. Line layers contain information on several related points (e.g. streets or borders). Polygon layers describe areas, e.g. administrative areas such as city districts or postcode areas. Examples of information that can be provided via polygon layers include regional coverage rates with doctors ..." (ThiBen et al., 2017, p. 1440).

Statistical analyses can then be used to establish correlations and visualise *spatial patterns*. Spatial patterns correspond to what is commonly referred to as thematic or functional maps, which are to be seen in contrast to geographical or political maps. "One example of an application for this are so-called 'heat maps', which illustrate complex data in a way that is easy to understand even for non-experts. These maps depict the dependent values of a two-dimensional definition set as colours or as a colour gradient (e.g. temperature) in addition to the geographical component (e.g. map). The colour gradient is based on the temperature distribution and runs from blue (e.g. cold) through green, yellow and orange to red (e.g. hot). The visualisation is used to intuitively capture particularly striking values in a large amount of data." (ThiBen et. al., 2017, p. 1440-1441)

2.2 Epidemiology and health services research as areas of application

Geographical research approaches and cartographic representations have existed in epidemiology since ancient times: "The spatial consideration of disease and health goes back a long way. Even Hippocrates investigated disease-ocological relationships between environmental conditions, lifestyle habits and human health." (Augustin et al., 2018, p. 629)

In German-speaking countries, the concept of medical geography was pioneered by the physician Leonhard Ludwig Finke, who described the first medical map towards the end of the 18th century. (Koller et al., 2020) August Hirsch, a German physician, epidemiologist and medical historian, published a three-volume handbook on historical-geographical pathology between 1859 and 1864. Another well-known historical example is the work "On the Mode of Communication of Cholera" by the English doctor John Snow from 1854, who recorded the deaths on a map of the city during a cholera epidemic in London. This enabled him to identify the wells that supplied contaminated water and thus spread the disease. (Thiften et al., 2017) Snow is considered the father of map-based analysis in inductive disease causation research. (Augustin et al., 2018) Also in Great Britain, the pediatrician James Alison Glover underpinned his research in the 1930s with geographical visualisation tools and was thus able to prove that the numbers of tonsillectomies on children in different school districts differed considerably: While in some districts only one in ten children had their tonsils removed, in others one in two had surgery. (Smith, 2011, p. 342).

In healthcare research, the cartographic approach is much more recent: in the 1960s, the nephrologist John Wennberg (*1934) began to research

medical care at regional level in the USA, referring to the aforementioned Briton Glover, among others. (Smith, 2011) In 1973, he published
Wennberg and the epidemiologist Alan Gittelsohn published the study "Small Area Variations in Health Care Delivery". (Wennberg/Gittelsohn, 1973) Using the US state of Vermont as an example, the two showed that there were considerable differences in care provision and medical infrastructure that were neither intentional nor planned and could not be explained medically.

With this and other works, Wennberg became the world's leading expert on undesirable deviations in the healthcare system. He later launched the Dartmouth Atlas of Health Care (TDI, 2023), which was first published in 1996 in the wake of the Clinton administration's failed healthcare reform (Smith, 2011) - at that time, of course, still in printed form. The work was financed by freed-up federal funds that had originally been earmarked for studies that were supposed to develop the basis for the reform. Under the impression of its failure in health policy, the Clinton administration made some of this money available to Wennberg to finance his hitherto grave project. The result was an eye-opener for the American public and painted a less than charming picture of the US healthcare system: "The original atlas showed, for example, a twofold variation in numbers of hospital beds, a threefold variation in numbers of doctors, fourfold variation in rates of coronary bypass surgery, and eightfold variation in radical prostatectomy. Importantly, more hospitals and doctors did not mean better outcomes." (Smith, 2011, p. 342).

Politicians at the time were less enraged by the injustice of the system, which was clearly evident in the unequal distribution of care capacities and services. Rather, they were particularly enamoured by the potential savings they saw in view of this unequal distribution of resources. Wennberg also provided figures: "The first atlas calculated that if every region in the country was like Minneapolis, then 120 000 beds could be closed and $32.6bn (£20.2bn; €23.2bn, at current exchange rates) saved without any deterioration in outcomes." (Smith, 2011, p. 342)

Today, the atlas is an extensive internet platform with maps and publications on the US healthcare system, which is also filled with the help of geoinformation systems. Smith compares its significance with the epoch-making work "On the Origin of Species" by Charles Darwin: "Both books resulted from a rigorous accumulation of data and fundamentally changed our world view. Darwin's book showed our descent from apes. The atlas exploded the belief that medicine is based firmly on science." (Smith, 2011, p. 342).

2.3 The growing influence of supply atlases

The Dartmouth Atlas was subsequently the inspiration for numerous projects in Europe, Australia and New Zealand. In 2010, for example, the NHS Atlas of Variation in Healthcare (NHS, 2023) was published in the UK based on its model. This provided the National Health Service with data that was considered revolutionary, "... for example, a near 30-fold variation in the percentage of patients in primary care trusts who receive all nine key care processes recommended for people with diabetes." (Smith, 2011, p. 342). Primary care trusts (PCTs) were the regional managing authorities of the NHS between 2001 and 2013.

Buhmann et al. identified twelve national supply atlases in Europe in 2018. Augustin et al. also identified 49 works with geographical presentation methods in Germany in 2018, of which they described 33 as "works with maps" and 16 as genuine "atlases". "The works differ, among other things, in the intended target group. It was found that the majority of the works considered here address two groups: on the one hand, the general public, such as interested laypersons, and on the other, multipliers, including journalists and teachers.

The smaller proportion of the studies found focussed on experts, which is evident, for example, in the preparation of the results." (Augustin et al., 2018, p. 630)

It is not only the number of care atlases that has increased in recent years, but also their importance in terms of their impact on real life. In the aforementioned study on the NHS Atlas of Variation in Healthcare, Schang et al. (2014) were able to show the extent to which it influenced regional decision-makers in the healthcare system: they analysed 51 of the 151 NHS PCTs at the time and found that 28 of them used the atlas to make decisions on investment or resource allocation. However, the authors also point out challenges for care atlases: "Publishing an Atlas of Variation may have great merit in stimulating the search and understanding of variations, but it may not be sufficient for achieving an impact on decision making about resource allocation." (Schang et al., 2014, p. 84)

In order to achieve this desired impact, the creators of such atlases had to overcome "generic hurdles" such as the limited availability of data and its lack of acceptance by decision-makers. However, once these hurdles have been overcome, a healthcare atlas can become a "tin opener" for the strategic planning of regional healthcare systems. And: "They may also help communicate strategic problems to clinicians." (Schang et al., 2014, p. 84). Ten years later, in the author's opinion, the problem with data is not so much its availability, but rather its linkability. In the healthcare system,

almost every major project encounters an interface problem at some point. This is also pointed out by the experts interviewed in the empirical part of this work.
As the number and influence of atlases increased, it also became necessary to introduce rules and guidelines for this research approach. In Germany, the guideline "Good Cartographic Practice in Healthcare" (GKPiG, Augustin et. al, 2017) has therefore been in place since 2017. In the author's opinion, this should also be followed in the future implementation of a cross-sectoral atlas of healthcare in the federal state of Salzburg, as the authors do not want to limit the content to Germany alone: "The addressees of these recommendations are all persons working in the healthcare sector, primarily from the disciplines of medicine, epidemiology, health services research, health economics or the public health service, who want to process health-related facts cartographically and have little geographical or cartographic expertise. The recommendations cover in particular the planning, preparation and creation of cartographic representations in the health sector. The GKPiG does not provide any advice on the interpretation of maps." (S. 8)

2.4 Focus on undesirable differences

As the example of the Dartmouth Atlas shows, modern medical atlases can no longer do without the support of geoinformatics systems. According to Thiften et al. (2017), the potential applications of such GIS can be divided into three areas:

1. Disease-ocological studies and presentations: How environmental influences affect the outbreak and spread of diseases is investigated and presented.
2. The presentation of risk factors: These can either have social causes (e.g. lifestyle or health behaviour), but can also be influenced by the environment (e.g. air or water pollution or noise).
3. Highlighting spatial and social differences in medical care.

While the first two points fall under epidemiology, the third area falls under health services research. For most examinations and treatments, there are regional differences in care. In most cases, these differences are justified and often even desired. For example, if a certain disease occurs more frequently in one region and therefore more examinations and treatments are necessary there than in others
regions. (Grote-Westrick, 2015). Wennberg's work was concerned with identifying and subsequently describing unwarranted variations. He defined these as "variation that cannot be explained on the basis of illness, medical evidence, or patient preference". (Wennberg 2010, p. 4) "Such unwarranted

variations must be identified and minimised, not only to improve the quality, fairness and cost-effectiveness of our healthcare system, but also and above all to avoid unnecessary stress, anxiety and danger to patients." (Grote-Westrick, 2015, p. 8)

In order to better summarise the differences, Wennberg developed three categories for the assessment of care structures and approaches. (Wennberg, 2010, Moen/Goodman, 2022)

- Effective care (effective or broadly effective care)
- Preference-sensitive care (preference-sensitive care)
- Supply-sensitive care (supply-sensitive care)

These categories also make it possible to categorise the causes of undesired differences: Effective care has more benefits than harms and brings about the desired outcome (Klempe- rer/Robra, 2014). As broadly effective care, it should be available to almost 100 per cent of the target population. This area includes screening programmes (Moen/Goodman, 2022) or, in Austria, examinations based on the mother-child pass.

Preference-sensitive care describes healthcare where there are either several possible indications or treatments or where a positive outcome is (still) poorly documented or controversial. This category can have massive effects, but also many causes: For example, regional differences in treatments in hospitals or in remote regions can reflect personal opinions or the strengths or weaknesses of doctors.

Categories for the assessment of care structures and approaches

Effective care (effective or broadly effective care)	*b* Affects only 1 5 to 25 per cent of all health services. *b* Has positive effects for those affected. *b* The care provides the desired outcome for the patients. *b* As broadly effective care, it is available to almost 100 percent of the target population - e.g. in the form of screening programmes.
Preference-sensitive care (preference-sensitive care)	*b* Affects up to 25 per cent of all treatments. *b* There are either several possible indications and/or treatments, or *b* a positive outcome is (still) poorly documented or controversial. *c* May also reflect personal opinions or the strengths or weaknesses of doctors. *b* Surgical specialists are particularly "susceptible" to preference-sensitive care. *b* May also reflect patients' cultural, social or political wishes or reservations (e.g. rejection of coronavirus vaccination).
Supply-sensitive care (supply-sensitive care)	*b* Affects 50 to 60 per cent of all health services. *b* Is dependent on resources such as free hospital beds, intensive care or available specialists.

Table 1: *Categories for the assessment of care structures and approaches - based on Wennberg (2010), Klemperer/Robra (2014)*

and Moen/Goodman (2022).

Surgical specialists are particularly susceptible to this category of regional differences. (Moen/Goodman, 2022). However, this may also be due to culturally or socially conditioned wishes or reservations of patients with regard to a treatment method (Klemperer/Robra, 2014). These wishes or reservations on the part of patients can be socially, culturally, religiously or even politically conditioned, for example. The fact that during the coronavirus pandemic in Austria, the population of entire communities or valleys was almost entirely unvaccinated is, in the opinion of the

The author provides a particularly vivid recent example of preference-sensitive care. Estimates assume that up to 25 per cent of all treatments fall into this category. (Wennberg, 2010)

Supply-sensitive care refers to medical services that depend on resources such as free hospital beds, available specialists or intensive care. Surgical specialists, but above all top medical specialities, are also particularly vulnerable in this area. This area accounts for between 50 and 60 per cent of all healthcare services (Moen/Goodman, 2022). And in the author's opinion, the importance of supply-sensitive care is likely to increase further as medicine becomes ever more specialised and technological.

Effective care thus describes the ideal state, which, however, only covers between 15 and 25 per cent of all care services and activities, while preference-sensitive care and supply-sensitive care carry an enormous "potential" of undesirable regional differences.

To summarise: The aim of health care atlases is to identify undesirable differences (Wennberg/Gittelsohn, 1973; Wennberg, 2010, Augustin et al., 2018) in health care and thus to show whether there is overuse or underuse in different specialities or regions. This has to do with ethics and justice on the one hand, but also with politics and economics on the other: undersupply provides political points of attack, oversupply shows possible savings potential (Smith, 2011; Buhmann et al., 2018). In contrast, epidemiological atlases are intended to show the regional distribution of diseases or symptoms, which can of course have an influence on care planning and management. In this respect, the boundaries between epidemiology and health services research are becoming blurred.

CHAPTER 3

3 best-practice examples for medical atlases

After important definitions, a brief historical overview of the state of research on geographical representations in medicine, the distinction between epidemiological atlases and health care atlases and the presentation of the purpose of health care atlases, three health care atlases are now presented that have repeatedly been positively emphasised in the literature (Smith, 2011; Mangiapane, 2014; Augustin et al., 2018; Koller et al, 2020) and can therefore be seen as examples of best practice. These are:

- the Dartmouth Atlas of Health Care (TDI, 2023 - www.dart-mouthatlas.org) from the USA,
- the health care atlas of the Central Institute for Statutory Health Insurance Physicians in Germany (Zi, 2023 - www.versorgung- satlas.de) and
- the cancer registry of the German federal state of Schleswig- Holstein (IKE, 2023 - www.krebsregister-sh.de).

3.1 The Dartmouth Atlas of Health Care

As described in the previous chapter, the Dartmouth Atlas of Health Care was first published in 1996 and fundamentally revised in 2007 for the then still young Internet age. The Trustees of Dartmouth College, which was founded in Hanover, New Hampshire, in 1769 and is thus one of the oldest universities in the USA, are listed as the media owners in the imprint. The Geisel School of Medicine, founded in 1797, is the medical school of Dartmouth College by Austrian standards. In 1988, John Wennberg founded the Centre for the Evaluative Clinical Sciences (CECS) - now the Dartmouth Institute for Health Policy and Clinical Practice - at the Geisel School of Medicine, which is the original sponsor of the Dartmouth Atlas. Wennberg was director of this institute until his retirement in 2007. (TDI, 2023)

Anyone expecting a clear, perhaps even interactive and constantly updated set of maps when they first visit the homepage www.dartmouthatlas.org will be disappointed. The home page is purist, showing a map only as the background of a content box and does not appear to be up to date at all, as the author points out in the news that the data from 2019 is now available for download in October 2023. Three content boxes refer to the "Research", "Explore" and "Understand" sections. Under "Research", there are extensive references to the data sources and an equally detailed description of the research method. Under "Understand", users are directed to collections of hundreds of reports and scientific articles (research articles), for which search functions are available.

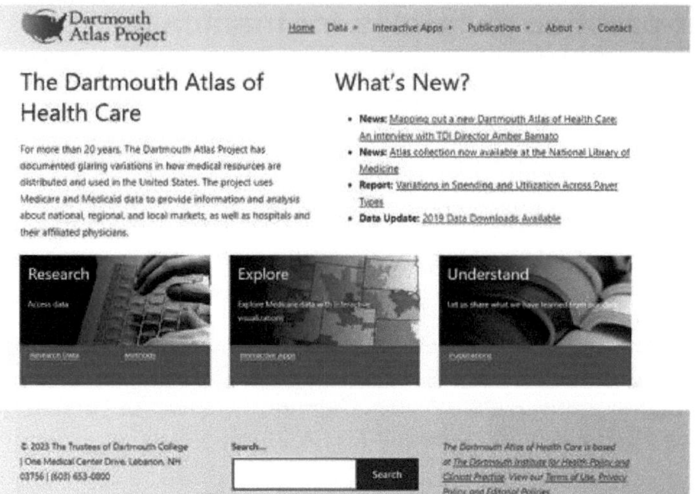

***Figure 1:** Home page of the Dartmouth Atlas of Health Care (https://www.dartmouthatlas.org) - accessed on 24 October 2023.*

The atlas thus also essentially consists of his large collection of scientific publications on various medical topics, which, although they all contain geographical

Many of them, however, do not contain a single map. An atlas in the sense of the definition used here can be found in the "Explore" section, which offers "Interactive Apps" on various topics - e.g. End of Life Care, End of Life Cancer Care, COVID-19, Primary Care Access, Surgical Discharges ... On the homepage of the interactive apps, users will find a tutorial with diagrams and a YouTube video explaining how to use the interactive cards.

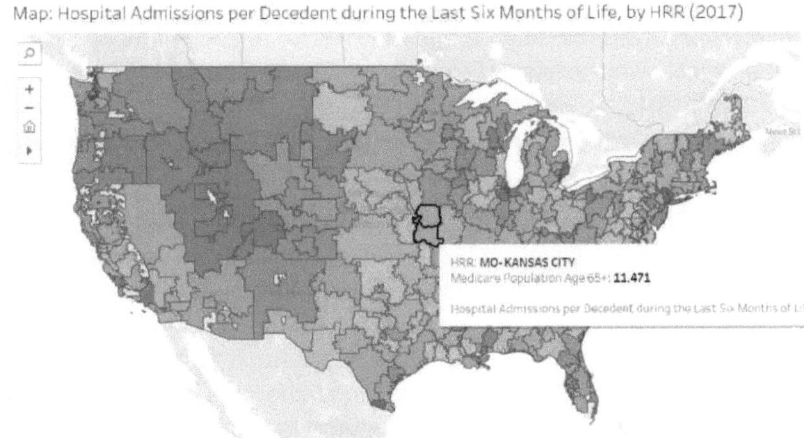

Figure 2: *Hospital admissions of deceased patients in their last six months of life with the Hospital Referral Regions (HRR; https://www.dartmouthatlas.org) filter - accessed on 24 October 2023.*

Each card has an introductory text that explains what it is about and establishes a link to the general theme of the Dartmouth Atlas: identifying undesirable differences in healthcare. On the subject of end-of-life care, it says: "The intensity of care in the last six months of life is an indicator of the propensity to use life-saving technology. The question of whether more medical intervention is better must be framed in terms of the potential gain in life expectancy for populations living in regions with greater intensity of intervention. Our research has provided evidence that populations living in regions with lower intensity of care in the last six months of life did not have higher mortality rates than those living in regions with higher care intensity." (TDI, 2023) Taking this abstract further, this means that there is apparently an oversupply of end-of-life care in individual regions of the USA, as the quantitative availability of the service does not have a positive impact on the desired outcome (life expectancy) of patients.

Specifically, in this example, the number of hospital admissions of deceased people in the last six months of their lives was calculated across the USA. Several filters/models are available for the maps: Hospital Service Areas (HSA), Hospital Referral Regions (HRR), Counties and States. HSAs and HRRs are the catchment areas of 3,436 local and 306 supra-regional hospitals. These two categories were developed by the Dartmouth Atlas team and published in the Atlas' extensive methodology section. The data for each individual unit can be viewed using a mouse-over function. The maps are displayed as heat maps and have a zoom function. In this example, which was accessed in autumn 2023, data is available for the years 2008 to 2017.

3.2 The care atlas of the Central Institute for Statutory Health Insurance Physician Care

In Germany, the Zentralinstitut für die kassenarztliche Ver- sorgung (Zi) offers a healthcare atlas, which can be found on the homepage www.versorgungsatlas.de. As the publisher, the Zi is registered in the imprint as the organisation responsible for the content and owner of the platform. This was founded in 1973 as a research institute, is based in Berlin and has the legal form of a foundation under civil law. The foundation is funded by the state associations of statutory health insurance physicians and the National Association of Statutory Health Insurance Physicians. The healthcare atlas was first published in 2011 and, unlike the Dartmouth Atlas, was designed for the internet from the outset.

Here, too, the start page is surprising - it contains neither a large picture nor a map, but is text-heavy with two graphics, each showing the outline of Germany - once embraced by a stethoscope and once on a globe held by a doctor in his right hand. The purpose of the atlas and the data sources are explained briefly: "The Health Care Atlas is a service provided by the Central Institute for Statutory Health Insurance Physicians in the Federal Republic of Germany (Zi) and offers information on medical care. The focus is on analysing and mapping regional differences. The analyses are based on the nationwide billing data for SHI-accredited medical care in Germany.[11] (Zi, 2023)

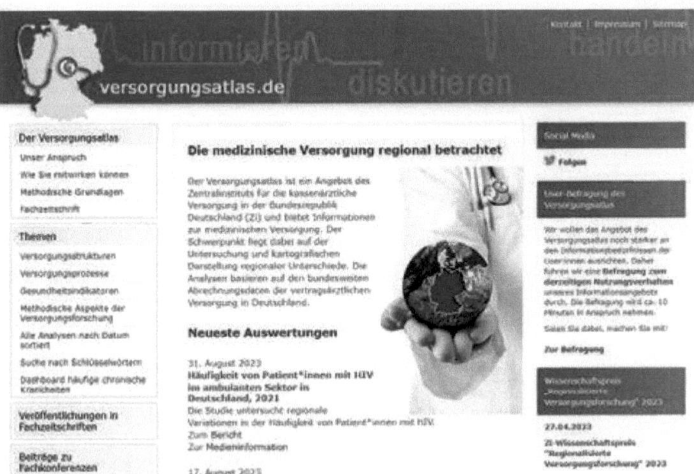

Figure 3: *The upper part of the homepage of the Zi Supply Atlas (www.versorgungsatlas.de) - accessed on 24 October 2023.*

The most important topics are summarised in content boxes on the homepage: Under "The Healthcare Atlas" you will find information on the scientific claim and the methodological basis. Users are also invited to participate. The topics include care structures and processes as well as health indicators. There is also a separate dashboard on common chronic diseases and links to scientific publications that have been produced in the context of the atlas.

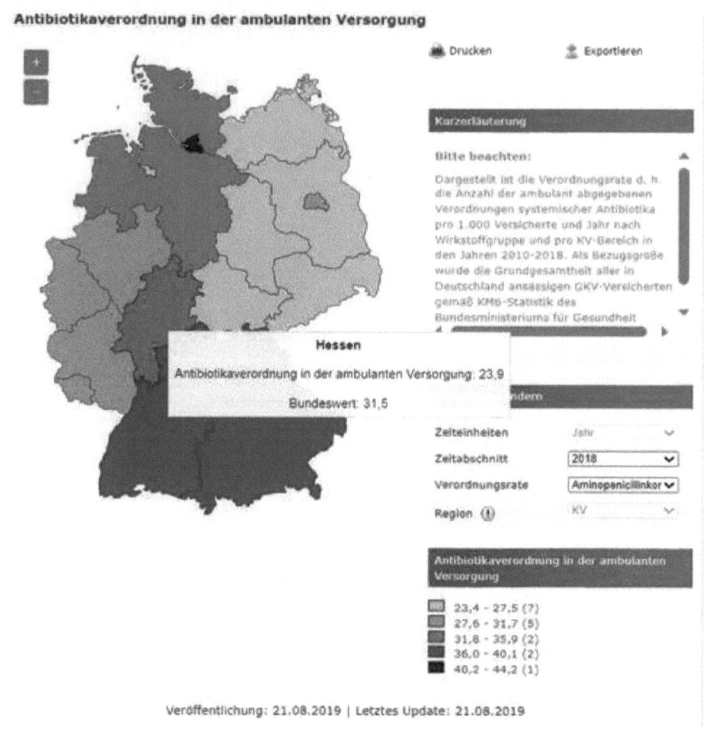

Figure 4: *Illustration of the number of antibiotic prescriptions in outpatient care per 1,000 insured persons and per year (www.versorgungsatlas.de) - accessed on 24 October2023.*

The maps relate to clearly defined topics and time periods - e.g. contract physicians and contract psychotherapists per 100,000 inhabitants by specialist groups and regions for the years 2014 to 2018 (published on 13. 09. 2019), specialist internists per 100.000 inhabitants - basic report 2011 (published on 10 March 2011), development of outpatient antibiotic prescriptions in a regional comparison - basic report 2008 - to 2012 (published on 6 October 2014) or nationwide incidence trends of diagnosed heart diseases in the years 2013 to 2021.

The maps are also designed as heat maps and are interactive. In most cases, only one federal state view is available - only North Rhine-Westphalia is subdivided into the regions of North Rhine and Westphalia-Lippe - and in a few cases a view at the level of the independent cities and districts. This means that most of the results are presented from a relatively high "flight altitude". In some cases - e.g. the map on the uptake of influenza vaccinations among chronically ill people from 2009 to 2019 - the data for individual federal states is missing. However, it is possible to track the development over several years. And in the example shown in Figure 4, the prescribed antibiotics are divided into ten categories, which provides interesting information for experts.

3.3 The Schleswig-Holstein Cancer Registry

The cancer registry for Germany's northernmost federal state is a web platform that was published for the first time in 2016 and contains an extensive cartographic representation. The trigger for the publication was the legal obligation for the federal states to set up clinical cancer registries:
"These [clinical cancer registries] collect and analyse data on the occurrence, treatment and progression of all cancer patients treated in the respective federal state. They thus provide the basis for quality assurance and research." (IKE, 2023)

Since 2016, doctors in the federal state have been obliged and at the same time authorised by their own state law, the Schleswig-Holstein Cancer Registry Act,
"to report a treated or investigated cancer, including precursors and early stages, neoplasms of uncertain and unknown behaviour and benign tumours of the central nervous system to the Schleswig-Holstein Cancer Registry". (IKE, 2023)

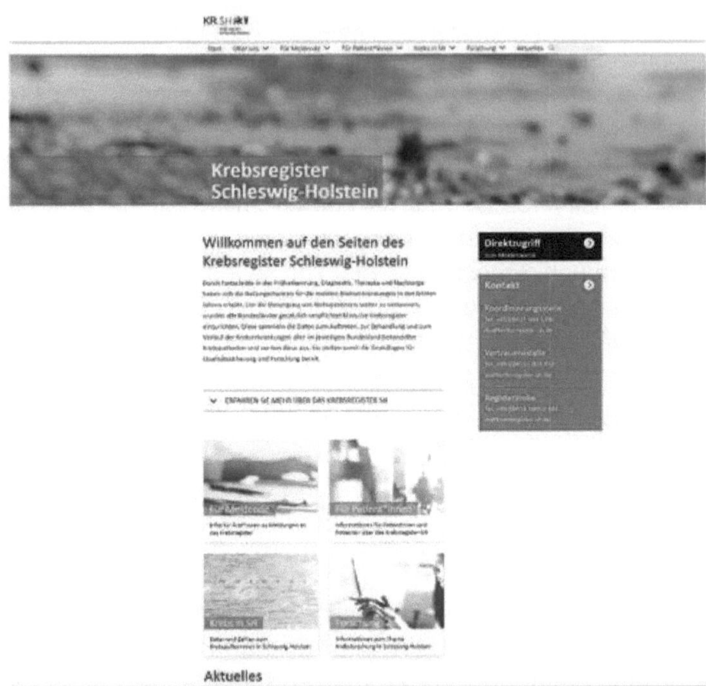

Figure 5: *The upper part of the homepage of the Schleswig-Holstein Cancer Registry* (www.krebsregister-sh.de) *- accessed on 25 October 2023.*

The imprint lists the Institute for Cancer Epidemiology (IKE) at the University of Lubeck, which is a public university and a foundation under public law. The homepage www.krebsregister-sh.de is visually characterised by a large-format photo of a pebble beach. A short information text is followed by content boxes that lead to the sections "For reporters", "For patients", "Cancer in SH" and "Research". These sections can also be found in the main menu above the feature photo. Links to current news about the Schleswig-Holstein Cancer Registry are listed below. Although the atlas was only published for the first time in 2016, the data goes back to 2006 in many cases and is updated annually.

In the "Research" section, the scientific community is offered opportunities to utilise data. In addition, reference is made to our own ongoing research projects as well as to international projects in which the Schleswig-Holstein Cancer Registry is involved or which it supports. There is also a clear list of scientific publications that have been written about the cancer registry, categorised by year. In the "For patients" section, patients are also offered the opportunity to participate in research projects (clinical studies) - an information sheet for downloading informs patients of their rights.

The central section is the interactive report, which is characterised by many tables, graphics and maps. It presents data and analyses on the 28 most common cancers. "General data is presented with an overview of incidence and mortality, the age distribution of incidence and mortality, incidence and mortality over time and in comparison with the figures for Germany as a whole. Furthermore, the prevalence by age is shown, absolute and relative survival by gender and tumour stage as well as information on some clinical parameters such as histology, localisation, tumour size, grading, etc." (IKE, 2023)

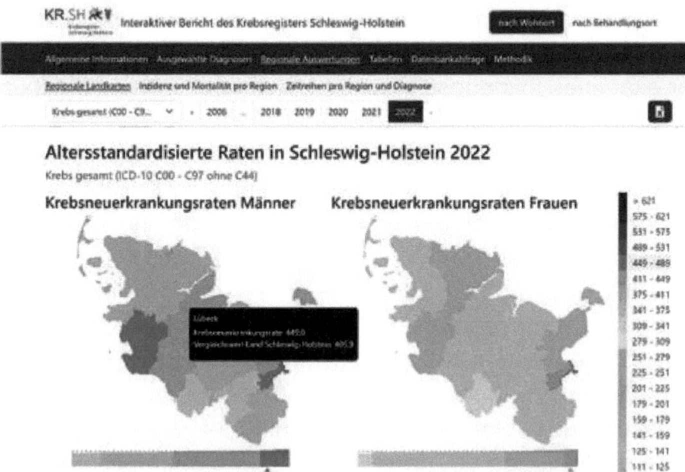

Figure 6: *Illustration of the new cancer incidence rates of women and men in Schleswig-Holstein for 2022 (www.krebsregister-sh.de) - accessed on 25 October 2023.*

The maps can be found under "regional analyses" and are shown at the level of the eleven administrative districts and four independent cities. They are also shown as heat maps in this atlas. A mouse-over function allows the data for the districts and independent cities to be viewed at a glance. As the maps were created looking back to 2006, it is also possible to visualise the development of cancer incidence.

The three best-practice examples presented are taken up again in the discussion. A checklist for a good care sat- las will be developed from the findings from the literature and the examples.

CHAPTER 4

4 Methodological comments and study design

4.1 The strengths of qualitative research and Interviews in health reporting

Following the preparation of the theoretical foundations of medical atlases in general and healthcare atlases in particular, the empirical part of this master's thesis is now concerned with developing the content-related foundations for a regional, cross-sector healthcare atlas for an Austrian federal state. As mentioned at the beginning, the central research question is: **How should a regional, cross-sector atlas of healthcare provision be structured for an Austrian federal state and what opportunities and challenges arise from its implementation?** As mentioned several times, the author examines this question using the federal state of Salzburg as an example.

To answer this question, he opted for a qualitative approach. Kelle/Tempel (2020) point out that qualitative research is not only suitable in the social sciences, but especially for the area of health reporting - in the author's opinion, a cross-sectoral health care atlas for the federal state of Salzburg clearly falls into the area of health reporting. In contrast to quantitative research, qualitative research does not aim to test precisely formulated hypotheses to see whether they can accurately describe relationships and thus predict outcomes. Qualitative research should depict reality and thus help to make predictions. At the beginning of the research process, categories are developed on the basis of general theoretical assumptions, for which data is then collected.

"The *data* is not collected in a standardised way using special measuring instruments, but through "open procedures", the results of which are less structured text data (such as written conversations, personal observation protocols), images or video recordings.

are. This data is not analysed using statistical methods, but through *interpretative* and *category-forming* procedures with the aim of identifying overarching patterns." (Kelle/Tempel, 2020, p. 1127 - emphasis in original)

To put it in the language of medicine: Qualitative research can be compared to the medical history taken by a doctor. One or more possible diagnoses are derived from the anamnesis, from which the indication and therapy options are then derived. Researchers who use qualitative methods derive one or more hypotheses from their data, the significance of which can then be investigated using quantitative methods.

Interviews are a frequently used qualitative research method. The author also decided to conduct interviews with experts and is in good company: "Expert interviews are used in a wide variety of research fields, often as part of a mix of methods, but also as an independent method" (Meuser/Nagel, 1991, p. 441)

Expert interviews are not about presenting the person with their orientations and attitudes in their living environment, but rather: "The context in question here is an organisational or institutional context that is not identical with the living context of the persons acting in it and in which they only represent a 'factor' ... Whether someone is addressed as an expert depends primarily on the respective research interest. Expert is a relational status. Expert status is in a certain sense conferred by the researcher, limited to a specific research question." (Meuser/Na- gel, 1991, pp. 442-443)

The author conducted interviews with "his" experts using an open guideline, as recommended by Meuser/Nagel:

"In our studies, we worked with open guidelines, and this seems to us to be the technically clean solution to the question of how to collect data. A guideline-orientated interview does justice to both the researcher's thematically limited interest in the expert and the expert status of the interviewee ... "Even if this may sound paradoxical, it is precisely the guideline that guarantees the openness of the interview process. By working with the guideline, the researcher familiarises herself with the topics to be addressed, and this forms the basis for a 'relaxed', unbureaucratic conduct of the interview." (Meuser Nagel, 1991. p. 448). Kelle/Tempel (2020) also point out the advantages of qualitative guided interviews. These are characterised by an openness that enables the interviewees to develop their own perceptions and perspectives during the interview.

4.2 Study design

Qualitative research methods are time-consuming. Interviews take much longer than answering a questionnaire, for example, and analysing them also requires significantly more time. (Kelle/Tempel, 2020) Therefore, only a limited number of interviews can be conducted for qualitative research. However, generalisability in the statistical sense of representativeness is also not the aim of qualitative research. Nevertheless, when selecting interview partners, care must be taken to ensure that as many aspects of the research area as possible are covered and that there is a balanced distribution of genders - of course only if the topic allows this. For example, in a qualitative study on the topic of what psychological pressure pregnant women feel exposed to, interviewing men would not seem to make much sense. Specifically, the author was guided by the following considerations:

- Stakeholders of the regional healthcare system in Salzburg are to be interviewed, as well as
- other experts from the regional healthcare system in Salzburg and from research.
- At the same time, both the gender distribution and the
- take into account the various fields of activity in the institutionalised healthcare system.

The author chose eight interviews with people who had the following affiliations:

- **Interview 1, hospital:** Decision-maker from the intramural sector. This is the largest and by far the most expensive area of the healthcare system.
- **Interview 2, administration:** decision-maker from the health administration.
- **Interview 3, social insurance:** Decision-maker from the field of medical care financiers. Specifically, a person from the area of social insurance was sought so that this area is also covered.
- **Interview 4, SHI-accredited doctor:** Representative of doctors in private practice with a health insurance contract. The owners of private ordinances were deliberately excluded here. Although private practices now have an influence on healthcare provision that should not be underestimated, they are not connected to the public healthcare system either institutionally or in terms of data technology in the same way as practices with health insurance contracts.
- **Interview 5, Nursing:** Representative of the nursing profession. Nursing is by far the largest professional group in the healthcare system. A person from the extramural sector was sought here. Although the number of carers in the intramural sector is greater than in the extramural sector, the person from interview 1 is already a representative of the intramural sector.
- **Interview 6, Pharmacy:** Representative of pharmaceutical care. In the author's opinion, too little attention is often paid to this when it comes to supply issues. Specifically, the author was looking for the owner of a pharmacy, as they have the greatest overview of the supply situation.
- **Interview 7, patient representatives:** Representative of patients' interests,
- **Interview 8, Research:** Research representative.

The interviews are cited in the results section with the above-mentioned designation. When preparing the study design, the author assumed that the number of eight interviews would be sufficient to achieve the necessary theoretical saturation (Merkens, 2009). The research process showed that this assumption was correct.

The author started the interviews with eight categories that had been deductively created in advance according to Kuckartz (2016). These categories were also the cornerstones of the interview guide, which is shown in the appendix. Their order did not imply any judgement, but rather followed a logical flow of conversation. At the beginning of the interview, the interviewees were informed that the possible foundations, content and challenges for a regional, cross-sector atlas of healthcare provision were to be developed using the example of the federal state of Salzburg. For this reason, only a regional atlas for Salzburg was mentioned in the course of the discussion.

- **Usefulness:** How useful does a regional, cross-sector atlas of healthcare provision in the federal state of Salzburg generally appear to be? What purpose could it fulfil from a meta-level perspective?
- **Scope of the content:** Should a cross-sectoral Salzburg Health Atlas only serve health services research or should it also cover epidemiological topics or answer questions?
- **Target groups:** Which target groups should be addressed?
- **Form of realisation:** Should such an atlas be designed as a written report or digitally or digitally and interactively? Should it be developed step by step - with a basis at the start and further modules in subsequent steps?
- **Content for the launch (must-haves):** What content or functionalities should such an atlas definitely offer at go-live?
- **Possible additional content (nice-to-haves):** Which content or functionalities should or could be implemented in the course of further steps.
- **Exclusion criteria (no-gos):** What content or functionalities can such an atlas not offer or perhaps should it not offer at all?
- **Stumbling blocks:** What major hurdles or challenges could arise during implementation?

CHAPTER 5

5 Results: Inputs from experts

Experts on a cross-sector care atlas for Salzburg

For this study, the author conducted a total of eight interviews with experts from the regional healthcare system in the province of Salzburg - four women and four men were interviewed between November 2023 and January 2024. The conversations all took place face to face - the author made audio recordings and transcribed the interviews afterwards. The interviews were analysed on the basis of a qualitative content analysis according to Mayring (2015); the categorisation system is based on Kuckartz (2016). The transcripts and coding sheets are available to the author for seven years from the date of publication and can be viewed on request. The analysis resulted in the following eight main categories with up to four sub-categories:

- **Category 1: "Meaning and purpose"** - with the sub-categories "Significance for society, healthcare system and science" and "Goals to be achieved".
- **Category 2: "Content"** - with the sub-categories "Scope of content" and "Projects to be included".
- **Category 3: "Target groups".**
- **Category 4: "Form of implementation"** - with the sub-categories "Technology" and "Organisation".
- **Category 5: "Must-haves to get started"** - with the sub-categories "Legal and organisational", "Content or function" and "Technology".
- **Category 6: "Nice-to-haves in further operation"** - with the sub-categories "Content", "Technology" and "Supporting measures".
- **Category 7**: **"No-Gos".**
- **Category 8: "Stumbling blocks"** - with the sub-categories "Legal and systemic", "Project level", "Data" and "Target groups not reached or depicted".

The paraphrased inputs (Mayring, 2015) of the experts on these main and sub-categories are presented point by point below and discussed and evaluated in the next chapter. A collated table with the paraphrased inputs can be found in the appendices to this thesis.

5.1 Category 1: "Sense and purpose"

Results category 1: "Sense and purpose"

Significance for society, the healthcare system and	***S*** Atlas provides new insights.
	S Atlas unearths previously unused treasure trove of data.
	S Atlas presents the healthcare system without taboos.
	e Atlas helps to ask questions and answer questions.

science	***U*** Atlas supports networking in the healthcare system. ***Γ*** Atlas is a guide for experts and health-competent citizens. Atlas helps to manage patient flows. Atlas helps to keep people in the healthcare system in basic care for as long as possible and thus relieves the burden on outpatient clinics. ***S*** Atlas contributes to the best possible outcome with the least possible effort.
Aims achieved	***S*** Atlas provides stakeholders and the population with a low-threshold overview of care structures. ***S*** Atlas identifies supply shortages and under- or oversupply. ***S*** Atlas takes into account the forecast population development. ***S*** Atlas is the basis for forward-looking planning of supply structures and required resources. ***S*** Atlas contributes to the fair distribution of services among system partners. ***S*** Atlas enables evaluation of decisions on supply structures. ***S*** Atlas presents current and future necessary care structures for common diseases ("widespread diseases"). ***S*** Atlas offers patients several options.

Table 2: *Results of category 1: "Sense and purpose"*

This category essentially corresponds to phase 2 of the interview guidelines. The author's aim was to ascertain whether the experts generally consider a regional, cross-sectoral atlas of healthcare to be useful, what "deeper meaning" such an atlas had in their view and what meta-goals it should pursue and achieve.

5.1.1 Significance for society, the healthcare system and science

The interview partners were unanimous in their opinion that a regional, cross-sector atlas for the province of Salzburg should definitely be implemented. It is seen as a suitable means of presenting the regional healthcare system clearly and quickly. In this regard, the experts currently identify deficits "because there is too little data available on the state of health and what needs to be done" (interview 6, pharmacy, 6-7). "There needs to be a proper, reliable database and data veracity." (Interview 2, administration, 7). In this sense, a regional health and care atlas could provide new insights.

The experts emphasise that although a lot of data is available on the (regional) healthcare system, this data is currently hardly linked to each other. (Interview 2, Administration, 155-157). Geographical processing of health data would help to uncover this unused treasure trove of data, as "you can simply recognise a lot through such representations that you cannot see purely from tables and data collections". (Interview 8, Research, 64-65). In this sense, a regional, cross-sector atlas of healthcare provision is also seen as a "very innovative tool" that "should be [available] in addition to all [other] current possibilities in the federal state" (Interview 7, patient representatives, 6-7). Such an atlas could also be the pilot project for a later nationwide solution. And it could serve as a source of data to underpin one's own positions in negotiations with the federal government: Salzburg's interests could be better represented "if we know where the shoe pinches in our own state, where the needs are". (Interview 2, Administration, 20-22).

A regional care atlas also makes sense because it could support better networking between stakeholders, providers and employees in the healthcare system: "My idea is that it improves collaboration and networking." (Interview 4, panel doctor, 10). The atlas could also serve as a guide through the healthcare system for both experts and patients and in this sense contribute to advancing health literacy overall (interview 5, nursing, 289-293).

The experts also consider a regional, cross-sector medical care atlas to be useful in light of the discussion about full hospital outpatient departments. The hope associated with such an atlas is that it could contribute to "keeping as many people as possible at the grassroots level" (Interview 3, social insurance, 176) and thus relieve the burden on outpatient clinics. The atlas could also help to ensure that "I bring out the best for the patient with the least possible effort" (Interview 4, SHI-accredited doctor, 12-13). In order for this to be possible, however, the atlas must illuminate all sectors "sufficiently and relentlessly" (interview 3, social insurance, 5).

5.1.2 Objectives pursued

At the meta-level, the experts cite two main goals and aspects: Firstly, a regional, cross-sector care atlas should provide both the general public and experts with an overview of the care structure that is accessible using common technology and therefore low-threshold (interview 2, administration, 61-53; interview 7, patient representatives, 193-216; interview 4, panel doctor, 22-27; interview 5, nursing, 14-16). This enabled him to make patients aware of the treatment options available to them. (Interview 4, SHI-accredited doctor, 47-60).

Secondly, it should be available as a planning tool for politicians, healthcare administration and the management of healthcare providers. It must therefore also identify current gaps in care and any overprovision and take into account the forecast development of the population. It could also help to "distribute the service business among the system partners ... ... according to capacity possibilities" (Interview 2, administration, 38-39) and to form priorities. The aspect of necessary forward-looking planning was emphasised by several interview partners - e.g. in Interview 1, Hospital (5-8): "The history of the last many, many decades has taught us that what has been done in the past may have fitted in once for the past, but we should finally take the long view and not do an RSG [Regional Structural

Plan for Health] in the rear-view mirror."
On the subject of forward-looking planning as a deeper meaning, it was also mentioned that the atlas could provide important information "to take the right actions" (interview 2, administration, 59) and also to identify planned or planned measures as not appropriate or not useful and thus prevent them. This requires a "common picture with the system partners" (interview 2, administration 60). In addition, a regional, cross-sector atlas of healthcare provision would also help to evaluate decisions made on care structures. "Control and planning. And really in a management cycle, which means that I set up the atlas, draw my conclusions, make sure that I reach the conclusions and when I have reached them, I see whether the care is what I want it to be." (Interview 3, social insurance, 36-39).
Since a regional, cross-sectoral care atlas should also take into account the forecast population development, it was possible to deduce from it which disease patterns - in this context the word "widespread diseases" was used (Interview 2, administration, 54; Interview 8, research, 68) - the healthcare system will be increasingly confronted with in the future and which structures must therefore be established or maintained for the future.

5.2 Category 2: "Contents"

Results category 2: "Contents

Scope of the In ha lts	**e** atlas depicts intramural and extramural structures down to municipal level. **e** Atlas covers acute and long-term care as well as prevention and aftercare (rehabilitation facilities). Atlas shows which diseases are to be expected in which age groups. **e** Atlas shows whether treatments are being carried out on time. ***n*** atlas is divided into sections for experts and laypersons. (male and female patients). ***S*** Atlas also offers contact options for the recorded structures.
Projects to be included	***S*** Population forecast of the state statistics. ***S*** Study "Paracelsus 10,000". ***J*** ELGA ***S*** SALK survey on demographic trends and hospitalisation rates.

Table 3: *Results category 2: "Contents".*

This category essentially reflects phase 3 of the interview guidelines. The author's aim here was to determine the scope of content that a regional, cross-sectoral supply atlas should have. The sub-category "Projects to be included" emerged during the evaluation of the interviews.

5.2.1 Scope of the content

With one exception (interview 1, hospital), there is a consensus among the experts that such an atlas should fully depict both intramural and extramural care structures. "It would really do both areas, intramural and extramural, a lot of good if there was an overview: What is available where?" (Interview 5,

Pflege, 6-8) The presentation was to be made down to the level of the 119 towns and municipalities in the province of Salzburg. "For me, the municipality would be the unit in such a care atlas - the district would be very, very rough." (Interview 8, Research, 40-41). In addition, according to some experts, not only acute care facilities, but also those for pre- and aftercare (e.g. rehabilitation facilities) should be taken into account. However, it has not yet been asked whether these representations should already be included in the first go-live of such a system. For all facilities, the contact details of the recorded structures or facilities should also be available in the atlas.

As already described in category 1 "Meaning and purpose", the atlas should not only depict the existing structures, but also serve as a planning, control and evaluation tool. Some experts therefore suggested dividing the atlas into sections for experts and laypersons or patients: "There should be two sections ... Everyone has a different perspective, of course, and that must be kept separate." (Interview 7, patient representatives, 10-12).

For the area of control/planning/evaluation, a regional, cross-sector atlas should also show which disease patterns occur more frequently in which age group or are to be expected in the future. Here too, it has not yet been determined whether this feature should be available at the first go-live. In addition, the aspect of timely care was brought into play in connection with the evaluation: "It's exciting to say that I'm getting the best quality pancreatic surgery for a pancreatic carcinoma. But if I don't get it for another year, I'll be dead from metastasis," was the pointed way the social insurance representative put it. (Interview 3, social insurance 71-73).

5.2.2 Projects to be included

Specifically mentioned here were the analyses of the Salzburg state statistics on the existing and expected population structure of the state. This would enable or provide "forecasting procedures and thus planning" as well as "better facts for prevention" (Interview 8, Research, 35-37). The data for this is available down to the municipal level and for the city of Salzburg down to the district level (Interview 8, Research, 40-43) and was probably also made available by the state of Salzburg for a regional, cross-sectoral supply atlas.

Two of the experts (interview 1, hospital, 43-50; interview 3, social insurance, 182-190) named the "Paracelsus 10,000" study as the central project to be included. This is currently the largest epidemiological study in Austria and is being carried out by Salzburg University Hospital. The aim is to "scientifically analyse the state of health of the Salzburg population to a high standard. In this way, diseases can be linked to age, origin and other

demographic data. These findings help to better understand and prevent the most common diseases and their origins." (SALK, 2023).
A randomised, representative sample of 10,000 people from Salzburg aged between 40 and 69 was included in the study. The first part was completed in March 2020 with the examination of the 10,000th test person. In the second part of the study, all test subjects will be invited to follow-up examinations. These will take place five
years after the first study phase. "Very good and valid results can be derived from the Paracelsus 10,000 Study as to how the state of health of the Salzburg population is developing." (Interview 1, hospital, 47-49)
A regional, cross-sector atlas of care structures also had to be coordinated with ELGA, as the electronic health portal already collates and provides a lot of data. (Interview 2, administration, 149-151). Another project to be included was a study by Salzburg University Hospital, which analysed the effects of demographic developments on the frequency of hospital admissions at the Christian Doppler Clinic campus. In summary, the figures show that in connection with neurological, neurosurgical and psychiatric treatments, increased hospitalisation is to be expected from the age of 45 and then from the age of 75. (Interview 1, hospital, 69-73).

5.3 Category 3: "Target groups"

Results category 3: "Target groups"
S Key target groups are decision-makers from stakeholders in the healthcare system and patients. However, the data is accessible to all interested persons (experts and laypersons).

Table 4: *Results category 3: "Target groups".*

This category essentially reflects phase 4 of the interview guidelines. In this phase, the author wanted to find out which groups of people a regional, cross-sectoral care atlas should be aimed at and which people or groups should use it. There is a broad consensus among the experts that the atlas should be aimed at two central target groups: 1. decision-makers from the stakeholders in the healthcare system as well as professionals from the healthcare sector.

the healthcare system; 2. patients. "I think it's relatively divided: One is the patient application, the other is for politics, for planning." (Interview 6, pharmacy, 135136) Although it was not specifically mentioned in the interviews, the author assumes that patients also refers to the parents of children and adolescents as well as the adult representatives or carers of people with disabilities. In addition to doctors and carers, the term "specialist staff" also includes therapeutic professions such as physiotherapy, occupational therapy, psychotherapy and speech therapy. (Interview 4, SHI-accredited doctor, 39-46). It was also important for some experts to note that the data must also be accessible to all interested persons - experts as well as laypersons. "I can't imagine an exclusion system because it wouldn't be consistent. Everyone gets the data if they want it." (Interview 3, social insurance, 144-147)

5.4 Category 4: "Form of realisation"

Results category 4: "Form of realisation"	
Technology	✓ ***Atlas is a digital, interactive platform with cartographic representations.*** ✓ ***Atlas differentiates between the target groups of stakeholders and patients.*** ✓ ***Reports and scientific articles on individual topics complement Atlas.*** ✓ ***Results are available for downloading and printing.***
Organisation	✓ ***The sponsor is a public or scientific institution.*** ✓ ***Financing is provided by public funds.*** ✓ ***Atlas has fixed human and financial resources.*** ✓ ***Atlas starts with limited content and is then expanded.*** ✓ ***Fixes team is constantly gathering feedback, expanding, updating and maintaining Atlas.***

Table 5: *Results category 4: "Form of realisation"*

This category covers phase 5 of the interview guide. The author's aim here was to ascertain how the experts envisage the implementation in broad terms - the sub-categories "Technology" and "Organisation" emerged during the evaluation of the interviews.

5.4.1 Technology

There was a consensus among the interview partners that the implementation of a regional, cross-sectoral healthcare atlas should definitely be digital: "The atlas also needs to be updated and kept up to date". (Interview 4, SHI-accredited doctor, 78-79) However, the wish was also expressed to provide printout options. The haptic was "more pleasant in certain areas" (interview 8, research, 112). Older people in particular need to be taken into account here: "Personally, I am still someone who would like to have a print version. I liked to have it [the result] on the table. I might also want to make a note of it." (Interview 7, patient representatives, 61-63) The possibility of download functions is also seen as necessary.

The experts are also unanimously of the opinion that it should be as interactive an online platform as possible with corresponding usability, whereby there should be cartographic representations as well as tabular lists and supplementary reports - see also the next category.

Reference was also made here to the different needs of the two main target groups: Experts and patients. For the experts, more in-depth figures, data and facts should be available, for which there could possibly be their own, reliable approaches. (Interview 1, hospital, 110-113). In this context, what was already mentioned in category 3 "Target groups" is emphasised once again: The basic information of a regional, cross-sectoral care atlas had to be accessible to everyone.

5.4.2 Organisation

The experts interviewed emphasised the conviction that not only the development and go-live of a supply atlas should be considered from the outset, but also its continued operation. A permanent team is absolutely necessary for this, which regularly updates the atlas, is the point of contact for queries of all kinds and should continuously obtain feedback on the forms of presentation, content and functionalities. (Interview 1, hospital, 178-183; Interview 2, administration, 199-201; Interview 5, nursing, 258-264; Interview 7, patient representatives, 193216). Specifically, it is emphasised in this context that not only the establishment, but also the operation requires "sufficient time, personnel and money". (Interview 5, nursing care, 260-261).

For the experts, it is completely open to discussion that a regional, cross-sector atlas must be supported by a public or scientific body. The Office of the Salzburg Provincial Government (interview 5, care, 150-157), the Paracelsus Medical University (interview 1, hospital, 178-183; interview 8, research, 241-250) and a new structure yet to be created (interview 2, administration, 197-208) were mentioned here:

- In the office of the Salzburg state government, an Altas should not be located directly in the health department. The overlaps between health and social affairs are fluid. Nevertheless, the topics are located in different political and administrative departments - "and it is an open secret that there are different sensitivities". It would therefore be "totally fine if there was a group that could go across both departments, so to speak". (Interview 5, nursing, 156-157).
- With regard to the PMU, the Research and Innovation Centre (FIZ) for Public Health and Health Services Research was specifically mentioned. (Interview 1, hospital, 178-183).
- The representative of the administration put forward the idea that a new publicly owned structure might need to be created in the regional healthcare system "to drive digitalisation issues forward" (interview 2, administration, 206-207). An atlas could then also be organisationally located in this structure. How this structure could be organised and who its

sponsors are was not discussed in any further detail.
As the sponsor should be a public or university organisation, the experts are in agreement that the funding must come from public funds. In general, "the stakeholders" or "the state" were named as funders.
The experts are also overwhelmingly of the opinion that the atlas should go online as a quick win (interview 2, public administration, 27-28) with predefined but limited content that has been agreed between the stakeholders. "I am an absolute advocate of organic growth," one expert put it in a nutshell (interview 3, social insurance, 75). Only one expert was of the opinion that "the big throw would be the right thing" (interview 4, health insurance doctor, 97), as only this would guarantee the credibility and thus acceptance of the project. However, there should be a trial run with test groups beforehand. Before the go-live, however, the system must "function properly, otherwise it will very quickly be the case that nobody uses it". (Interview 4, SHI-accredited doctor, 105106).

5.5 Results category 5: "Must-haves for the start

Results category 5: "Must-haves for the start"

Law and Organisation	Clear will of the necessary stakeholders: Provincial politics, administration, hospitals, social insurance providers and professional organisations.
	V Self-help groups, senior counselling services and representatives of inpatient and outpatient long-term care provide input. Atlas fulfils scientific requirements.
	e awareness of ethical responsibility - data can lead to the reorganisation or dismantling of structures.
	S Valid data is also available for the future.
	S Cooperation agreements also secure data flows for the future.
In ha lt or function	***u*** Atlas provides an overview of all intramural and extramural structures down to municipal level.
	u Atlas presents existing and future care structures for cardiovascular diseases, diabetes and brain health.
	a Atlas provides contact details of the care structures.
	S Feedback to the Atlas team is possible.
Technology	***S*** Atlas displays the data geographically.
	S Atlas offers a search function with filter options.
	S Atlas offers download and print functions.
	S There are processes for ongoing updates.

Table 6: *Results category 5: "Must-haves for the start".*

This category represents phase 6 of the interview guide. In this part of the interviews, the author wanted to find out what the experts believe are the prerequisites for a go-live of a regional, cross-sector supply atlas. The sub-categories "law and organisation", "content or function" and "technology" also emerged from the evaluation of the interviews.

5.5.1 Legal and organisational

The experts interviewed agreed that there must be a clear commitment from the stakeholders involved for the implementation of such an atlas. The following stakeholders were named as necessary: Provincial politics and administration, hospitals, social insurance providers and professional organisations - specifically the Chamber of Physicians and the Chamber of Pharmacists. "There must be the political will, but also the will of those who have the data. Otherwise it won't work." (Interview 8, Research, 171172) Experience from earlier, unspecified projects has shown that it makes sense to secure this clear commitment through cooperation agreements. (Interview 8, Research, 168171).

Agreement should also be reached with the representatives of the therapeutic professions and nursing, even if these professional groups are less tightly organised than doctors and pharmacists. (Interview 6, pharmacy, 180-197) To this end, the Chamber of Commerce was also brought on board as the legal representative of freelance therapists. (Interview 2, Administration, 189-191). In addition, it was also suggested that representatives of self-help groups, senior counselling services and organisations for outpatient and inpatient long-term care should be asked for input during the development and for feedback on ongoing operations.

When asked about must-haves, it was also emphasised that a care atlas must fulfil scientific requirements. (Interview 1, Hospital, 13-19 and 113-119; Interview 8, Research, 196-200). A regional, cross-sectoral care atlas should also not be limited to a one-off snapshot. It is much more important to ensure that the flow of required data is legally and organisationally secured from the outset. This is where the aforementioned cooperation agreements come into play. (Interview 8, Research, 155-162). The aspect of "high responsibility" (interview 3, social security, 338) associated with such a project was also mentioned. This is because it is also the task of the atlas to identify gaps in supply or oversupply, which could lead to resources (having to) be redistributed.

5.5.2 Content and function

For this area, it has already been shown in category 2 "Content" that the experts are of the opinion that a regional, cross-sectoral care atlas should provide an overview of all intra- and extramural structures down to the municipal level in one part - including contact information. In another part, the atlas should also present treatment pathways for common clinical pictures - in this context, as already mentioned, the term "common diseases" or "contemporary diseases" was used (Interview 3, social insurance, 85). Specifically, three disease groups should be started with: cardiovascular diseases, diabetes and brain health (stroke care). (Interview 1, hospital, 13-19 and 77-81; Interview 2, administration, 54-55; Interview 3, social insurance, 85-87). Functionally, the atlas should be technically structured in such a way that users can give the care team low-threshold feedback.

5.5.3 Technical

It is undisputed among the experts that it makes sense to map the care structures. However, as there are so many available services - in some cases more than 100 at municipal level alone (interview 5, care, 278-286) - a search function with filter options had to be available - tailored to the target group of experts and laypersons. (Interview 3, social insurance, 294-318; Interview 4, general practitioner, 110-132; Interview 7, patient representatives, 10-14; Interview 8, research, 112-118). The

Search results should be able to be printed out or downloaded. The download function is also needed so that reports on detailed topics can subsequently be derived.

It was also emphasised that long-term operation and later modular expansion should already be worked towards when creating the atlas. "You shouldn't think small, you should think very holistically and include all factors that affect the location. And it makes sense to start rolling out the whole thing on a pilot basis with individual [modules]." (Interview 2, administration, 103-104) Due to this long-term requirement, processes for updating data should *not* only be secured legally, but also technically. (Interview 8, Research, 155162)

The experts agree that a regional, cross-sectoral care atlas must be updated on an ongoing basis in order to be useful and accepted. The individual interviewees had different views on what "ongoing" actually means. The intervals mentioned were "annually" (interview 1, hospital, 120-124), "every six months" (interview 7, patient representatives, 109-111), "quarterly[11] (interview 5, nursing, 271-277) and even "continuously" (interview 8, research, 196-200).

5.6 Results category 6: "Nice-to-haves in further operation"

Results category 6: "Nice-to-haves in further operation"

Contents	***A*** Atlas visualises patient flows. Information brochures for patients are produced on the basis of the atlas. ***A*** Atlas regularly provides up-to-date reports on specialised topics. ***A*** Altas provides information on the functions and tasks of the healthcare professions. ***A*** Atlas contains information about apprenticeships and vacancies. ***A*** Atlas contains tips for self-help. ***A*** Atlas presents complementary social offers.
Technology	***A*** Atlas is available as an app for mobile devices. ***p*** Atlas has advanced search and filter by symptoms. ***A*** Atlas offers ticket system for enquiries.

	A Atlas offers appointment co-ordination or jumping-off points for appointment co-ordination. ***A*** reports are also available as podcasts.
Accompanying measures	***A*** The atlas is widely advertised. ***A*** There are terminals at public places as access points to the atlas. ***A*** The establishment of medical group practices is being promoted. ***A*** The non-medical extramural sector is being expanded. ***A*** Pharmacies are increasingly integrated as part of the healthcare system. ***A*** There are peers or guides through the healthcare system at local level. ***A*** Prevention, health promotion and self-help are strengthened. ***A*** The health literacy of the population is required. ***A*** Financial flows in the healthcare system are simplified. ***A*** The payment system is changed from the performance principle to the success principle.

Table 7: *Results of category 6: "Nice-to-haves in further operations"*

This category reflects phase 7 of the interview guidelines. The author's aim here was to find out what functions and content a regional, cross-sector supply atlas should have, but does not necessarily have to have when it goes live. The sub-categories "Content", "Technical" and "Flanking measures" emerged from the evaluation of the interviews. In the third sub-category, general wishes or ideas for a reform or further development of the healthcare system were summarised, which were expressed by the experts, but only very marginally or had nothing to do with the actual topic of the work. Nevertheless, the author has decided to include these points because the results chapter would be incomplete without them.

5.6.1 Contents

It has already been explained in the previous categories that a regional, cross-sectoral care atlas should depict care structures down to the municipal level and have patients and experts as central target groups. For further operation, the wish was also expressed that such an atlas should also depict the actual patient flows, i.e. it should show which doctors or other healthcare providers people go to with which problems - meaning both the local and the content-related dimension. So is the decision to go to the outpatient clinic the result of a lack of services in private practice or an expression of greater trust in intramural care? (Interview 1, hospital, 152-157).

It was also suggested that the data collected in the atlas could be used to create information leaflets that could be "handed to someone when they are discharged from hospital and said: Look, this is what the route looks like if you have any questions". (Interview, 6, Pharmacy, 79-81) In general, further reports or reports on special topics could also be derived from a care atlas. (Interview 1, hospital, 138-145; Interview 3, social insurance, 179-182; Interview 7, patient organisation, 112-117).

For the (prospective) employees or trainees in the healthcare system, the atlas could serve as an information platform about training and further education opportunities in the federal state or even about available training places. (Interview 2, Administration, 111-113)
The content on intramural and extramural care services was subsequently supplemented by information on social (counselling) services. "Especially in the extramural area, the dividing line between the social area and the health area is often not clearly recognisable." (Interview 5, nursing, 91-93) And in terms of improving the health literacy of the Salzburg population, an atlas could also provide information about the functions and tasks of the health professions and contain tips for self-help, e.g. household remedies for colds or instructions for treating minor wounds. (Interview 5, Nursing, 91-102 and 167-172).

5.6.2 Technology

The desire for an app version for smartphones was also expressed in the interviews. This could also offer interviews and reports in the form of podcasts. (Interview 7, patient representatives, 112-117) An extended search function would also be conceivable, in which the relevant contact points could be found by entering symptoms, as well as a system through which the public could make enquiries about health issues. Tickets were automatically created for each enquiry, which were then processed by a pool of experts. A nationwide system for booking health appointments online would also be desirable. This system could be integrated directly into the atlas or the atlas could be a jumping-off point for such a booking system. (Interview 5, care 91-102 and 175-189).

5.6.3 Accompanying measures

It was noted as an important accompanying measure that the atlas should be widely publicised so that it is accepted by the experts, but above all by the population. (Interview 5, care, 264-266; Interview 8, research, 144-154). The desire for terminals or access points in public places, e.g. in municipal offices or squares, where people could access the care atlas directly, also goes in this direction. This was compared with information systems such as those found in large shopping centres. (Interview 5, Care, 110122).
The need to promote the establishment of group practices and primary care facilities in the province of Salzburg was also emphasised. (Interview 3, social insurance, 240-254, Interview 6, pharmacy, 167-176). On the one hand, this would be in the interests of the employees of the healthcare system, but on the other hand, it would also be a significant improvement for patients, as it would make it possible to extend opening hours in the extramural sector.

It was repeatedly noted that the services offered by the nursing and therapeutic professions also needed to be mapped in a care atlas. In general, these non-medical extramural services should be expanded, especially in rural areas. "If you are a man somewhere in a Flachgau community, are bedridden and have an indwelling catheter, then you have a problem. There are only a few GPs left who make house calls. And you need a GP who comes every six weeks to change the catheter." (Interview 5, Nursing, 228-231)

Pharmacies are also important points of contact with the healthcare system for the population. There, people could ask experts questions directly. Conversely, pharmacies were often not perceived as important healthcare facilities. The knowledge and expertise available there is currently still underutilised. Pharmacies should therefore be more closely involved. (Interview 6, pharmacy, 60-69 and 269-274)

Overall, the aim of health policy and administration should be to provide the population with better health education. This would be possible, for example, through the introduction of peers or guides at local level, who would guide (newly) affected patients through the healthcare system or introduce them to it after acute events, for example. To prevent this from happening in the first place, some experts believe that prevention, health promotion, self-help and health awareness should be strengthened. "We need to finally raise awareness among the population: Hey, it's not my GP's diabetes, it's my diabetes and I have to deal with it." (Interview 5, nursing, 320-321) However, all of this requires better overall health literacy among the population (Interview 5, nursing, 177-191, 211-216, Interview 6, pharmacy, 255266).

At the same time, the financial flows should also be simplified - "the most sensible solution would be to place all payments in one hand" (Interview 6, Pharmacy, 151-152). And one could even think about completely reorganising the healthcare system financially - away from the current performance principle, in which payment is essentially based on the treatments provided, towards a success principle that pays healthcare providers for maintaining people's health. (Interview 5, Care, 293-326).

5.7 Results category 7: "No-Gos

Results category 7: "No-Gos"
✓ Atlas establishes links between clinical pictures and patients' ethnic origin, religion or sexual orientation.
✓ Atlas pursues economic interests.
✓ The pharmaceutical industry is a key partner of the Atlas.

✓ Churches and religious communities are integrated into the atlas.

Table 8: *Results category 7: "No-Gos"*

This category essentially corresponds to phase 8 of the interview guidelines. The author's aim was to determine what content or functionalities a regional, cross-sector atlas of healthcare should not or perhaps must not offer. In terms of project management, these are therefore the non-objectives.

In addition, ethical requirements were specified that had to be adhered to in any case. Misuse of the information or data had to be ruled out in any case. (Interview 8, Research, 97-104). For example, one interviewee warned against "drawing any ethnic or other conclusions" - for example in connection with "skin colour, origin and religion". These aspects should "in any case be left out" (Interview 1, hospital, 168-171). In addition, "economic interests naturally had to take a back seat" (interview 5, nursing, 89). For this reason, pharmaceutical or medical technology companies should not play a role in the development and operation of such an atlas: "I would be careful with pharmaceutical companies because I believe that they should not penetrate too deeply into the state healthcare system." (Interview 6, Pharmacy, 190-191).

Religious aspects should also be excluded as far as possible, although the Catholic Church as the operator of religious hospitals,
care homes and mobile support services plays an active role in the healthcare system. "I am in favour of a separation of church and state." (Interview 6, Pharmacy, 195). Fundamentalist religious communities and sects should at best be viewed against the background that dropouts could become patients in need of mental health care. For example, Salzburg now also has its own self-help group for people who have left cults. (Interview 7, patient representative, 89-94, 142-148).

5.8 Results category 8: "Stumbling blocks"

Results category 8: "Stumbling blocks"	
Legal and systemic	✓ ***Changes in the healthcare system and demographics are not taken into account.*** ✓ ***Too little consideration is given to data protection and data security.*** ✓ ***Ownership rights to the data are not taken into account.*** ✓ ***Lack of commitment on the part of stakeholders/carriers - also for the future.*** ✓ ***Important stakeholders are not on board.*** ✓ ***Different (financial) interests of stakeholders.*** ✓ ***Providers of oversupply feel attacked.*** ✓ ***There is resistance from political parties and professional***

	organisations. ✓ ***The population knows too little about the healthcare system, e.g. the GP system or the purpose of emergency admissions.***
Project level	✓ ***The project is planned too big.*** ✓ ***The meaning and purpose of the project are communicated too little or unclear.*** ✓ ***Budget and personnel are not secured for the future.*** ✓ ***Key objectives and promises are not being fulfilled.*** ✓ ***Too much data leads to confusion.*** ✓ ***The focus - presentation of the data - is lost, technology becomes an end in itself.***
data	✓ ***Data is not up-to-date, incomplete or not robust.*** ✓ ***There are too many data sources.*** ✓ ***Data cannot be integrated due to missing interfaces.*** ✓ ***Data generation effort does not justify the result. Evaluation of data generation is missing.*** ✓ ***There is no standardised understanding of how to interpret the data.*** ✓ ***Data is transferred with incorrect interpretation - subsequent error.*** ✓ ***Processes for data generation and data transfer are not secured for the future.*** ✓ ***Data is not available for all participants.***
Target groups that cannot be reached or are not depicted	✓ ***The elective doctor sector is currently under-recorded.*** ✓ ***People from educationally disadvantaged backgrounds and with a migration background are difficult to reach.*** ✓ ***Many people, especially older people, have no or only poor internet access.***

Table 9: *Results of category 8: "Stumbling blocks"*

This category is essentially reflected in the ninth and final phase of the interview guide. However, the interviews quickly revealed that aspects of this category were mentioned in all phases of the dialogue. The sub-categories emerged during the evaluation of the interviews. Some inputs were repeated in the interviews, e.g. "must-haves" and "stumbling blocks" - in the sense that if a must-have is missing, this jeopardises the success of the project.

5.8.1 Legal and systemic

From a meta-level perspective, the project of a regional, cross-sector atlas is doomed to failure if it only updates the past and present, but does not take into account the "very strong change" in the healthcare system (Interview 4, GP, 163-164). However, it was left open how this change should be taken into account in concrete terms.

Legal aspects were mentioned in connection with data aggregation,

management and interpretation. "The topic with the
We always have data protection." (Interview 5, nursing, 16) Under no circumstances should a health atlas lead to glassy-eyed patients (Interview 6, pharmacy, 240-250). In addition, it was necessary to regulate or record which institution owns which data and which groups of people have the right to read or further utilise which data. (Interview 8, research 164-165, 213-215).

Systemic stumbling blocks are the lack of central partners or irreconcilable differences in interests. Several interviewees pointed out these aspects/dangers. (Interview 1, hospital, 19-25, 159-164; Interview 2, administration, 155-162; Interview 6, pharmacy, 215-226, Interview 7, patient representatives, 173-178, Interview 8, research, 204-206, 209-213). Specifically, the Medical Association was mentioned here as a necessary but structurally conservative professional organisation that does not give up "anything without a fight". (Interview 6, Pharmacy, 213). The aspect of diverging party-political interests was also mentioned, but only in passing. (Interview 3, social insurance, 230-235; Interview 8, research, 209-213). The economic aspects played a greater role. Above all, if the atlas revealed overprovision in individual areas, the dismantling of structures that are not necessary from an economic point of view could lead to massive resistance from the sponsors of these structures. (Interview 3, social insurance, 330-336).

5.8.2 Project level

According to the experts, many critical mistakes can be made in this area. For example, project plans that are too ambitious or a project scope that is too large can lead to failure (interview 2, administration, 156-157; interview 3, social insurance, 45-59). "As soon as you make it too big and complex, there is a very, very high risk that it will fail." (Interview 8, research, 183184) An atlas that is too complex and extensive would lead to confusion and ultimately to the project not being accepted. It was also important to ensure that the focus - the easily understandable preparation of data on the healthcare system - was not lost sight of. IT technology should not become "an end in itself". (Interview 8, research 191-196). At the same time, it was emphasised that despite a clear and focused project plan, it was important not to think small. (Interview 2, Administration 100-107).

It is also important for success that the key objectives and promises of a supply atlas are met. (Interview 8, Research, 177-186). At the same time, the deeper meaning and purpose of the project must be adequately communicated to the representatives of the stakeholders and the population. (Interview 6, pharmacy, 226-229). And the financial and human resources had to be secured in the medium to long term. (Interview 4, GP, 159-171) The atlas would probably need five years to get off the ground before it was recognised and valid in terms of content. (Interview 5, nursing, 26-28)

5.8.3 Data

Aspects relating to data have already been explained in several interview phases and categories. They are summarised here once again and the points indicated are explained in more detail here. The experts consider it critical for the success of the project that the processed or edited data must be up-to-date, complete and resilient in the sense of a critical discourse. "You don't need data, you need robust data." (Interview 3, social insurance, 240) At the same time, there should not be too many different data sources and data. (Interview 5, care, 278-286). The interfaces required to connect data from different sources are always an issue in IT projects. Such interfaces are sometimes very complex to programme. It is important to ensure that the effort justifies the result, i.e. the gain in knowledge. (Interview 8, Research, 164, 224-228).

A transparent system must be set up for the generation and aggregation of data, which technically enables continuous updating and is also continuously evaluated during operation. In the past, one-off data collections with "surveys and other aberrations" had often led to ambitious projects "getting stuck". (Interview 8, Research, 147155). Access to the raw data must be guaranteed for all participants, otherwise mistrust could arise. In addition, all sponsoring organisations of a regional, cross-sectoral care atlas had to agree on uniform interpretations of the incoming data and the data presented. "You need a proper database, reliable data and data veracity." (Interview 2, Administration, 7). Any system that combines data from multiple sources is prone to errors. "The trick will be to aggregate the data in such a way that I minimise the error that I will inevitably make - according to a Gauft curve." (Interview 3, social insurance, 252-254).

5.8.4 Target groups that cannot be reached or are not depicted

One possible stumbling block mentioned was that older, chronically ill people, as a key target group of a care atlas, could hardly be reached with a digital tool, as many older people either do not have access to the internet or only have a weak bandwidth. (Interview 7, patient representative, 180-184). However, another interviewee commented that the elderly should not be underestimated - the number of Internet users among them is increasing all the time. (Interview 6, Pharmacy, 88-89). It was also noted that people from less educated backgrounds or with a migration background are generally difficult for the public healthcare system to reach. "You can see that there is an absolute community problem." (Interview 3, social insurance, 198).

An important group of medical providers are the elective doctors, who provide around 50 per cent of care in the province of Salzburg, e.g. in the field of gynaecology. (Interview 3, social insurance, 621). However, elective doctors are currently barely covered by the public healthcare system. "When it comes to elective doctors, we're in a data fog." (Interview 3, social insurance, 262)

5.9 Summary

In summary, the following picture emerges from the expert interviews:

- The experts are unanimously in favour of setting up a regional, cross-sector care atlas for the federal state of Salzburg.
- According to the experts, this atlas must be digital and interactive.
- It is intended to address two central target groups: 1. decision-makers in the regional healthcare system and experts; 2. current and future patients and thus de facto the general population.
- Financing is to be provided by public funds.
- The atlas should provide knowledge and must fulfil scientific criteria.
- The sponsor should be a public or scientific organisation.
- The structure of the atlas should start with a few, precisely defined basic functions in the sense of "quick wins" - but further development should already be considered during the planning phase.
- The most important basic function is the complete, cartographically prepared representation of all intramural and extramural supply structures in the federal state. The 119 cities and municipalities of the federal state are to be seen as a unit - a finer "granulation" should be considered for the state capital.
- The treatment pathways for "common diseases" - specifically cardiovascular diseases, diabetes and brain health - will also be presented as a basic function at the launch.
- The atlas should also include the population forecast and existing epidemiological studies from the federal state of Salzburg and thus enable the planning and management of care structures.
- Without stakeholder commitment, the project is doomed to fail.
- Contracts between the stakeholders must ensure that valid and "robust" data that is accepted by all is available both during construction and operation.

CHAPTER 6

6 Discussion: What a cross-sector care atlas for the province of Salzburg should look like

So far, the literature and three best-practice examples have been used to illustrate what geographical visualisation methods can achieve in epidemiology and health services research. Interviews with experts show what opportunities, requirements, wishes and challenges there are for a regional, cross-sectoral health care atlas for the federal state of Salzburg. These results now need to be discussed.

6.1 Categories of medical atlases

In the author's opinion, medical atlases can be divided into four categories - see Table 10: 1. area covered (supranational, national, regional, local); 2. content (epidemiological atlas, health care atlas, mixed form); 3. target groups (experts, decision-makers, wider public); 4. form of implementation/preparation (analogue, digital or digital and interactive). The vast majority of publications that are labelled as medical atlases by their authors cannot be classified as such, even if the definition given in Chapter 2 is interpreted fairly. The few actual atlases are often hybrid forms - e.g. European atlas of ECMO care, national atlas of extramural and in-hospital care and the distribution of common diseases or regional atlas of dementia care. In most cases, the boundaries between care research and epidemiology are blurred.

Of the best-practice examples, the Dartmouth Atlas and the Zi Care Atlas are clearly categorised as care research. They have the declared aim of drawing attention to undesirable differences in care provision. Although Augustin et al. (2018) and Koller et al. (2020) see the Schleswig-Holstein Cancer Registry as a health care atlas, the author considers it to be an epidemiological atlas that only indirectly allows conclusions to be drawn about health care provision. This shows how blurred the boundaries are between epidemiological atlases and health care atlases.

The Dartmouth Atlas and Zi-Care Atlas cover entire state areas, while the Schleswig-Holstein Cancer Registry covers a single region. All three best-practice examples are digital and contain numerous interactive heat maps, although the Zi-Care Atlas usually only has a very large filter (the federal states). All three combine the components of software, hardware, data, methods and organisation, making them comprehensive geoinformation systems (Thiften et al., 2017).

Categories of medical atlases

Area covered	Form of realisation

✓ supranational ✓ national ✓ regional ✓ local	✓ analogue ✓ digital in report form ✓ digital with cartographic representations ✓ digital and interactive with cartographic representations
Target group(s) ✓ Experts ✓ Decision-makers and decision-makers ✓ wider public	Contents ✓ Epidemiological atlas Supply atlas ✓ Mixed form

Table 10: *Categories for categorising medical atlases - created by the author.*

In the author's opinion, the Dartmouth Atlas and Zi-Atlas are primarily aimed at experts and decision-makers: They use many technical terms that are not or only partially explained; despite the references provided Expertise is required to understand and interpret the tables. The Schleswig-Holstein Cancer Registry is also aimed at a broader public such as interested laypersons and multipliers such as journalists and teachers (Augustin et al., 2018) and has a separate section for patients. Overall, the language used is more bourgeois than that of the Dartmouth Atlas and Zi-Care Atlas. All three examples provide numerous scientific publications of their own. The Zi-Atlas team also invites external researchers to actively contribute in a separate section. In the Schleswig-Holstein Cancer Registry, the external participation of doctors is even prescribed by a separate state law.

6.2 What makes a good medical care atlas?

Let us now turn to what makes a good supply atlas - the author has identified four categories:

- Impartiality and acceptance,
- Scientificity,
- Relevance,
- User-friendliness and accessibility

Various sources (Mangiapane, 2014; Schang et al., 2014; Ulrich et al., 2017; Augustin et al., 2018; Koller et al., 2020) contain individual aspects that the author takes up here and supplements with his own considerations. This closes the knowledge gap identified in the first part. Table 13 summarises the criteria in the appendices.

6.2.1 Impartiality and acceptance

In the author's opinion, this point is essential for a good care atlas. It is no coincidence that the sponsors of the three best-practice examples shown are public research institutions: Universities are behind the Dartmouth Atlas and the Schleswig-Holstein Cancer Registry, while the Zi was founded as a research institute in 1973. It would be questionable if the sponsor of a medical atlas was a pharmaceutical company, a political party or an institution that is close to a political party, e.g. a think tank, an interest group or an association.

Furthermore, in the author's opinion, the editorial team should not be able to act without supervision. In the case of an atlas sponsored by a university or research institute, a scientific advisory board is a suitable supervisory body. In the case of regional corporations, this can be a parliamentary body or a body appointed by parliament, in Austria, for example, the Court of Auditors, and in the case of (public) corporations, a supervisory board.

In the author's opinion, impartiality and control are two essential prerequisites for acceptance; a third is publicity: the three best-practice examples are projects in the public interest that are predominantly publicly funded. The author does not consider it unethical per se to generate economic benefits from a medical atlas. However, this should not be the driving force, but only serve to refinance part of the costs for creation and operation.

6.2.2 Scientificity

A good health care atlas must primarily aim to gain knowledge: "The atlas primarily serves to describe and discuss spatial differences and to generate new hypotheses." (Augustin et al., 2018, p. 632) It goes without saying that reliability, validity and objectivity (Wolf/Best, 2010) as well as formal criteria such as correct citation and gender-appropriate language are adhered to - both in the cartographic representations and in supplementary reports and scientific contributions. In addition, the field (Mangiapane, 2014; Augustin et al.; 2018, Koller et al., 2020) refers to the following scientific guidelines:

- "Good Epidemiological Practice" (Hoffmann et al., 2014),
- "Good practice secondary data analysis" (Swart et al., 2015),
- "Good cartographic practice in healthcare" (Augustin et al., 2017),
- "Good practice in health reporting" (Starke et al., 2019).

In the author's opinion, a good care atlas complies with these guidelines.

6.2.3 Relevance

Relevance means that the content is substantive, meaningful and tailored to the needs of the target groups. This criterion is also based on the author's own considerations. Comments on this can only be found indirectly in the literature (Mangiapane 2014, Augustin et al. 2018, Koller et al. 2020). In order to achieve relevance, the author believes that data should be updated regularly - a requirement that the three best-practice examples fulfil. Interestingly, the author found no indication in the literature that a good atlas must be up to date.

Relevance also means benefit for the scientific community and/or decision-makers. Mangiapane (2014) emphasises that the declared aim of the Zi care atlas is to provide decision-makers and researchers with data and analyses on defined care issues and to discuss these publicly. Ulrich et al. (2017) also emphasise the need to involve (local) experts in the processing and presentation of regional healthcare data: "These experts know the existing healthcare structures best and can provide interpretation aids and point out special features that are not readily apparent from the data." (Ulrich et al., 2017, p. 1380)

All of the examples presented also provide detailed, ongoing reports, thereby developing the field as a whole. However, none of the atlases enable forecasting, for example by linking the expected population development with care data or epidemiological data. In the author's opinion, however, this would increase its relevance.

6.2.4 Accessibility and user-friendliness

In the digital age, accessibility means that a good medical atlas is available online without restriction. The preparation must comply with the generally recognised rules of usability. The content of the data must be presented clearly and comprehensibly - the aforementioned guidelines exist for this purpose. Textual accessibility has already been mentioned. A good online medical atlas must also be technically accessible as far as possible. This means that screen readers can read the texts aloud or that it is possible to use simple keyboard shortcuts and technical aids, as people with physical disabilities use on the computer. The Web Content Accessibility Guidelines (WCAG) of the World Wide Web Consortium (W3G, 2023), which have been recognised as ISO/IEC standard 40500:2012 since 2012, provide instructions. Since 2020, the European Union has stipulated that new websites of public bodies must fulfil at least the AA level and thus the middle of three levels of accessibility.

The author knows from his professional practice in the Salzburg regional hospitals that modern websites are not only barrier-free, but also follow the principle of "mobile first": First and foremost, the presentation must work on smartphones. 70 per cent of all

The Salzburg provincial hospitals' website is accessed via smartphones, with the remaining 30 per cent mainly being accessed by our own

employees. Interactive maps are reaching their limits. Nevertheless, the Schleswig-Holstein Cancer Registry essentially fulfils the requirements of responsive design: the maps adapt to the screen size and can also be used on small screens. The Dartmouth Atlas, on the other hand, does not show any maps in the mobile version and the presentation of the tables can be categorised as inadequate. In the desktop version, all three best-practice examples use heat maps, which visualise complex data in a way that is easy to understand even for non-experts (Thiften et. al, 2017).
User-friendliness also means that interpretation aids and information on limitations and interpretation errors are available (Augustin et al., 2018; Koller et al., 2020). For example, the editorial team of the Schleswig-Holstein Cancer Registry states that spatial differences can arise by chance and that similar spatial patterns alone do not mean a connection. It also points out that although large areas dominate the map, they are often sparsely populated and their significance is therefore overestimated. The editorial team of the Zi-Atlas in turn provides detailed discussions in all reports, as is customary in scientific contributions. These discussions are particularly emphasised by Augustin et al. (2014), as they point out limitations, offer help with interpretation and point out which correlations cannot be derived from the maps.
The author understands the four criteria of impartiality and acceptance, scientificity, relevance as well as accessibility and user-friendliness as a checklist that should be worked through when creating a cross-sector care atlas for the federal state of Salzburg. Subsequently, the results of the expert interviews are compared with the criteria of the checklist.

6.3 Impartiality and acceptance

The expert interviews show: There is no doubt that a regional, cross-sectoral care atlas makes sense, is publicly funded and must be supported by a public or scientific body. This raises two questions: Where should the funds come from? And which public body could this be?

6.3.1 Broad commitment vs. group of the willing

In 2023, Austria spent 50.8 billion euros on healthcare; this corresponds to 11.4 per cent of GDP. (Statistics Austria, 2024) 77.8 per cent comes from taxes and social security contributions, 22.2 per cent comes from private health insurance companies and directly from citizens. Various tax revenues are used to pay for mobile services and nursing homes as well as public hospitals. The five contributory social insurances (AUVA, BVAEB, OGK, PVA and SVS) cover the other part of the hospital costs as well as those for rehabilitation, extramural medical and therapeutic care as well as medicines and medical products. (Gesundheit.gv.at, 2024) Both the federal

government and social insurances are federally structured, which results in a complex financing system with federal and state funds and other structures.
Compared to total healthcare expenditure, a regional, cross-sectoral healthcare atlas for a federal state is a small project. However, most of the funds are tied up in the healthcare system - decision-makers have only marginal financial room for manoeuvre. There are therefore fierce battles in the public political discourse and within the organisations for the available financial resources. Added to this are the different interests of the stakeholders, which the experts also pointed out in the interviews, as well as traditional role models. In many conversations with doctors and pharmacists, for example, the author has witnessed the objections that one professional group triggers in the other.
It therefore seems sensible at first glance to ensure a broad commitment from all stakeholders before developing a regional, cross-sectoral care atlas for Salzburg. Specifically, these are:

- Province of Salzburg (politics and administration),
- Carrier of the public fund hospitals in the federal state,
- Social insurance institutions (umbrella organisation of social insurance institutions as well as OGK, SVS, BVAEB, AUVA, PVA)
- Medical Association,
- Chamber of Pharmacists,
- Chamber of Commerce (as the legal representative of the freelance non-physician healthcare professions).

In politics and administration, the decision-making authority lies in Salzburg. Currently, the provincial government includes the governor as finance officer and the provincial health councillor, whereby the financing of the healthcare system has been directly assigned to the health department since 2023. The social insurances have regional offices in Salzburg, but the strategic decisions are made in Vienna. The interest groups are organised federally - the regional organisations have more competences than the regional offices of the social insurances, but are bound by the federal policy. Conclusion: A broad commitment cannot be made in Salzburg alone. The author worked for several years in Vienna in leading journalistic positions (chief of staff, deputy editor-in-chief and editor-in-chief). During this time, he experienced how little importance regional political and health issues from the West East have in Vienna. In addition, there is a broad commitment to
In the author's opinion, this is only possible if financing and sponsorship have been clarified. Negotiating the distribution of costs could take months

or years and would tie up enormous organisational and economic resources.
The author therefore considers an alternative strategy to be more expedient: an implementation project should start in Salzburg with a group of willing people who agree on a quickly realisable project scope in line with the experts interviewed, but who also consider future expansions and provide for technical and content-related interfaces during development, to which further modules can dock in the future. Of course, this means restrictions, but these should be accepted in the interests of a quick win and a pragmatic, realis- tic approach. Further considerations follow in subchapter 6.5 "Relevance". In addition, self-help groups and representatives of outpatient and inpatient long-term care should be involved in an advisory capacity - as suggested in the interviews.
In terms of a quick win, one body should also make financial contributions in advance for planning and implementation in order to avoid lengthy financial negotiations at regional level. This can only be the state of Salzburg in the form of the health department - state politics and state administration have the greatest benefit of all stakeholders.

6.3.2 Existing scientific structures for a Realisation project

The client should be the entire state government in order to give the project the necessary political backing. In addition to representatives of the "willing parties", experts from the healthcare system and from research should also be involved in the realisation of the project and should take the scientific lead in its development. There are already structures in place that can be utilised:

- The IDA Lab (Lab for Intelligent Data Analytics Salzburg) is located at Paris Lodron University Salzburg (PLUS), "a competence centre for basic and applied research as well as for knowledge and technology transfer in the fields of data science, machine learning, AI and statistics. It is a cooperation between the Paris Lodron University of Salzburg (PLUS, project leader), the Paracelsus Medical University (PMU), the Salzburg Research Forschungsgesellschaft (SRFG) and the Salzburg University of Applied Sciences (FHS)". (PLUS, 2024) The state is calling for the IDA Lab as part of the Salzburg Science and Innovation Strategy 2025 (WISS 2025).
- Experts from the fields of medicine, nursing, pharmacy, health sciences, epidemiology and health services research conduct research and teach at the PMU. They form a scientific consortium that is formally organised in the Research and Innovation Centre (FIZ) for Public Health and Health Services Research. (PMU, 2024).

• There is also a Biomedical Data Science and Big Special Data research team at the PMU.

• As already mentioned several times, the scientific expertise of state statistics should be brought in from the state administration.

6.3.3 Possible carriers

In the author's opinion, the state of Salzburg should take the financial and organisational lead in setting up the atlas, but not the responsibility for day-to-day operations. This could lead to mistrust on the part of the other partners and would damage the acceptance and thus also the release. The sponsors of the best-practice examples are university institutions. What solutions were possible for Salzburg?

The public PLUS does not have a medical faculty and can therefore be ruled out as a sponsor from the author's point of view. One possibility would be to locate the Salzburg Health Care Atlas organisationally in the FIZ for Public Health & Health Services Research and thus at the PMU. However, the private sponsorship of the PMU by a foundation stands in the way of this. The federal states are legally and politically restricted in the financing of private universities, as there is also a public university system. However, the public sector can certainly pay for specific projects and services provided by private universities. This means that it must be ensured that the project financing of the Atlas *does not* become basic financing for the PMU. In the author's opinion, this can be solved by means of contracts. An advisory board made up of stakeholder representatives was able to guarantee the control that the author defines as an essential prerequisite for acceptance in the checklist for a good supply atlas.

As a second option for sponsorship, one expert mentioned a newly founded organisation in which digitalisation projects for the regional healthcare system could be bundled. (Interview 2, administration, 197-208) According to the author, a non-profit limited liability company could be founded for this purpose, in which the stakeholders hold shares. A supervisory board would be responsible for control. There had to be a clear demarcation between this company and the ELGA system to prevent duplication or competition. This would only require a clear project mandate.

Conclusion: Both the connection to the PMU and the foundation of a new organisation seem possible. From the author's point of view, however, there are more arguments in favour of using the existing structure of the FIZ for Public Health and Health Services Research. This is networked in the regional and (inter)national scientific community, which would make it much easier to integrate further qualified scientific work during operation, following the example of best-practice examples. A non-profit limited company, on the other hand, first had to build up the necessary scientific expertise and network within the community, which jeopardised acceptance, especially in the important start-up phase.

6.4 Scientificity

The author sees the fewest challenges in this area. The expert interviews have clearly shown that there is no doubt that a regional, cross-sectoral supply atlas must fulfil scientific requirements. However, some details should be clarified or taken into account when setting up the atlas.
For example, a statute should establish the scientific character and thus make it binding for all stakeholders. The author assumes no resistance here. Reliability, validity and objectivity are beyond doubt. Gaining knowledge as a central goal is also common sense. The fact that a supply atlas describes spatial differences in supply structures is due to the nature of the project. However, it must be taken into account that the scientific results will lead to political debates and distribution battles. However, this should not be an obstacle for the project per se.
There could be discussions about the scientific guidelines for action. The author mentions four German guidelines in the checklist. Can these be transferred one-to-one to Austria? Are adaptations necessary? Do own guidelines have to be created? As mentioned, the author is of the opinion that the guidelines should be adopted and, if necessary, interpreted in detail with regard to regional circumstances. After all, there are many internationally recognised guidelines and "good practices" in medicine and nursing that also apply in Austria.
The project idea itself also speaks in favour of adopting the German guidelines: if you look at the care atlas for Salzburg at the meta-level, it is about bringing together and visually processing existing data from the healthcare system. In May 2022, the EU Commission presented a draft regulation for the creation of a European Health Data Space (EHDS - Common European Data Spaces). Since December
In 2023, there will be a common position of the EU Council and thus of all member states. One of three stated goals: The EHDS "calls for the use of health data for better medical care, research and policy making" (European Commission, 2024). In this sense, the Salzburg Healthcare Atlas was a pre-fulfilment of a planned and already politically agreed EU regulation. So why should guidelines from the largest EU country be unsuitable for Salzburg?

6.5 Relevance

The atlas must provide the target groups with new insights. And to an extent that justifies the effort required to set it up and operate it. (Interview 8, Research, 164, 224-228) Although it is not the aim of this study to provide an estimate of the necessary human and technical resources, it is clear that the costs of setting up and operating a regional, cross-sectoral care atlas will be considerable. Ulrich et al. (2017) used the example of dementia care in the district of Gieften (Hesse, Germany) to investigate whether scientifically usable data is already available or can be collected for a small region and came to the following conclusion: "The example of small-scale care planning presented in this article shows that care-relevant data is available at a small-scale level, but that it can only be created and analysed with a relatively high personnel and financial outlay." (Ulrich et al., 2017, 1379) This statement is several years old, but still applies in the author's opinion.

6.5.1 Presentation of care services as the lowest common denominator

The expert interviews show: The lowest common denominator for the go-live content is the complete representation of all care structures in the federal state. The atlas is designed to provide professionals and the general public with a quick overview. Without going into technical and content-related details or usability tools such as search filters and graphical presentation, the author believes that this lowest common denominator can be realised with reasonable resources within a reasonable period of time. This lowest common denominator alone would provide a better overview than all currently available websites, regional structure plans, studies or other lists.

However, it is necessary to clarify what is meant by a complete representation of intramural and extramural care structures. For the intramural sector, the answer seems clear at first glance: we are talking about those public hospitals that are financed by SAGES (Salzburg Health Fund). Specifically, these are ten hospitals from five sponsors: Salzburg University Hospital with the Campus Landeskrankenhaus and the Campus Christian Doppler Clinic, the regional hospitals in Hallein, St. Veit and Tamsweg (all SALK), Oberndorf Hospital (VAMED), the UKH (AUVA), the Kardinal Schwarzenberg Clinic (Barmherzige Schwestern) and the Tauernklinikum with the sites in Zell am See and Mittersill, which is de facto owned by the two municipalities. It will be necessary to clarify how detailed the services offered by the hospitals are presented in the atlas. The author considers it sufficient to record the medical departments and their wards (with bed sizes) and outpatient clinics. Large hospitals and their capacities could be included right at the beginning, but also in a further expansion stage.

How do we deal with private clinics? This will require a fundamental decision by the stakeholders. One argument in favour of the private hospitals in the atlas is that they are relevant for the provision of care - especially in obstetrics, gynaecology, orthopaedics and traumatology. The same question also arises for the extramural sector. Should health insurance practices or those of elective doctors, therapists and midwives without health insurance contracts be covered? The current debates surrounding the sharp rise in the number of elective doctors show that this topic is relevant to professional and party politics as well as the media. One thing is clear: elective practices are an integral part of healthcare provision, as the experts in the interviews point out.

The author is of the opinion that an atlas would be incomplete without the inclusion of private clinics and elective practices, which would inevitably lead to a lack of acceptance. Therefore, the private sector should definitely be included. However, it is not possible to show how much private clinics and elective practices contribute to the provision of care in detail, as individual experts suggest. This is because private providers are not (yet) integrated into the systems of the public healthcare system and therefore do not have to document or prove which services they provide. An indirect determination of the volume of services - for example via opening hours, findings or private prescriptions issued - would completely contradict the principle that only valid, reliable data that is accepted by all parties involved should be included in the atlas.

Which extramural healthcare professions should be included at all? The study "Healthcare professions in Austria" (Weiss, et al., 2023) published by the Federal Ministry of Social Affairs, Health, Care and Consumer Protection can be used as a guideline here. In the author's opinion, the following occupational groups should be included if the persons concerned work directly with patients in an independent capacity or in a comparable constellation:

- Doctors (general practitioners and specialists),
- Dentists,
- Clinical psychologists,
- Health psychologists and health psychologists,
- Psychotherapists and psychotherapists,
- Music therapists and music therapists,
- Midwives,
- Advanced medical-technical services (physiotherapy, di- atology, occupational therapy, speech therapy, orthoptics),
- Health and nursing care (community nurses),
- Training therapy,

• Medical massage therapists and medical masseurs.

(Family) pharmacies and primary care units (PCUs) should also be recorded. A PVE entry should show which medical and therapeutic specialists the centre offers. In the author's opinion, professional organisations and the project group must inform individuals and facilities in advance that ...

• ... they are recorded in a supply atlas,
• ... this serves the transparency of the healthcare system,
• ... this also reveals possible over- or undersupply,
• ... they also (have to) supply data directly or indirectly (via specialist organisations).

The healthcare providers are registered in their respective professional registers or professional organisations. The aim is for all self-employed and established units (group practices, PVEs, pharmacies) to be covered. During implementation, it is important to check whether an obligation is desired or even legally possible.

According to the experts, the complete overview of the care structures, this lowest common denominator, should be available to everyone. In the author's opinion, the individual entries had to be linked to important, basic information: Is it a public hospital or a private clinic? Is there a health insurance contract for a practice? How can the user reach the facility by phone and/or e-mail? When is it open? From his experience as project manager of an internet reform of the Salzburg state hospitals, the author knows that a single point of truth should be the aim for websites: Information should only be entered once and then linked. Links to the respective homepages would ensure that the care atlas always provides up-to-date information.

In the author's opinion, two topics should be added to the lowest common denominator for the go-live. 1. biographical data from registered doctors, midwives, therapists and community nurses, which are available in the professional registers, should also be included. With just a few clicks, this would show who is due to retire and when. Of course, this personal data must be truncated, which means that the atlas must have a small protected area that is only accessible to the health administration and, to a limited extent, to experts. 2. the population forecast of the state statistics, which is available down to municipal level, should be included. All in all, this would result in a planning and control tool with a simplicity and quality that is unique in Austria.

6.5.2 Data jungle as the biggest challenge

Whether the treatment pathways for "widespread diseases" need to be

presented at the go-live stage, as several experts suggest, is a decision that must be made in an implementation project. After careful consideration, the author comes to the conclusion that the "widespread diseases" should be left up front at the start because he sees hardly any solvable challenges. For example, there is no centralised coding system in the extramural medical sector. This means that epidemiological representations based on valid, uniformly collected and generally recognised data are not possible in Austria. This was also the conclusion reached by the Austrian Court of Audit in an audit of healthcare provision during the first phase of the COVID-19 pandemic. The "lack of standardised diagnoses in the private practice sector" and the "time delays between the provision of services and billing" were cited as major problems. (Rechnungshof Osterreich, 2021, p. 19) The lack of a coding system means, for example, that it is impossible to collect the exact number of people with diabetes in Austria.
In addition, the entire area of elective practices is "data-heavy in the neighbourhood", as one interviewee put it (interview 3, social insurance, 262). For this reason, experts from the health administration have long been calling for elective doctors to be obliged to "use the e-card" and thus be linked to the social insurance information system, ELGA and a central coding system that is to be set up. "We need a proper, reliable database and true data," one expert demands (interview 2, administration, 7). It is currently not possible to trace the treatment pathways of "common diseases" on the basis of reliable data.
One could argue that other sources of data could be used and that statistical methods could produce useful results. In Austria, there is no shortage of sources for health data: Degelsegger-Marquez/Grubock/Fidon wrote the study "Health data in Austria - an overview" for Gesundheit Osterreich GmbH in 2022. It does not contain a single figure. Instead, the team of authors lists more than 40 pages of sources, where which institution collects which data and identifies "around 25" relevant federal laws. The metaphor of the data jungle is indeed appropriate. Recently, the COVID-19 pandemic has clearly demonstrated to politicians, administrators, the media and citizens the state of data quality and the connection of various data sources in the Austrian healthcare system. In the aforementioned report, the Austrian Court of Audit states "... that it was not clear to the federal government from which sources the states collected their data and which special features had to be taken into account in each case. There were also no specifications (e.g. on evaluation dates or the circumstances surrounding the survey)." (Austrian Court of Audit, 2021, p. 54).

6.5.3 Nice-to-haves: Supplementary reports and studies on the supply atlas

At best, in the author's opinion, the editorial team was able to publish additional studies parallel to the go-live on the burdens on the regional healthcare system that are to be expected in connection with the aforementioned "widespread diseases" for the various population cohorts. The projects mentioned by the experts are available as data sources: the population development projection, the "Paracelsus 10,000" study and the SALK survey on demographic trends and hospitalisation rates in connection with neurological, neurosurgical and psychiatric illnesses.
Such supplementary studies available at the go-live could serve as a benchmark for the further scientific handling of the care atlas. In the checklist for a good care atlas, the author states that the editorial team should regularly derive reports on special topics or invite external experts to publish such reports on the atlas platform. This point relates to further operation and should definitely be taken into account during the set-up phase, but from the publisher's point of view it does not represent a technical, content-related or political challenge. The only limiting factor for the editorial team is its size and financial endowment. The atlas could quickly become more relevant if academic theses were published in its context. This in turn speaks in favour of embedding it organisationally in a university environment.
All other nice-to-haves mentioned by the experts in the interviews are justified and can be implemented in further phases. With regard to the "accompanying measures", only the desire for broad advertising and for terminals in public places as entry points to the atlas are relevant to this topic. Both are tied to the financial framework of the project and therefore depend on the will of the stakeholders.

6.6 User-friendliness and accessibility

In terms of user-friendliness and accessibility, the experts provide many tips and express many wishes that are in line with the literature and best-practice examples. Clear and comprehensible visualisations are possible thanks to heat maps. High usability and interactive utilisation options such as zoom functions, search, search filters, scroll, mouse-over or download functions are standard. There are ready-made applications for feedback options - basically, it is sufficient to provide a central e-mail address.
However, a greater challenge - as the author knows from his professional practice - is the aforementioned linguistic accessibility. Many experts in the healthcare system have problems summarising data and facts in generally understandable language. For this reason, the editorial system of the

healthcare atlas should develop the expertise to translate experts into a language that is accessible to citizens. This citizen-friendly language should also be used for the comprehensible summaries, interpretation aids, references to limitations and possible interpretation errors required in the checklist.

CHAPTER 7

7 Summary

7.1 Summary

This work shows that the creation of a regional, cross-sectoral care atlas is in the interest of experts from various areas of the regional healthcare system in the province of Salzburg. It also shows that there are best-practice examples abroad at national and regional level on which a project in Salzburg can be based. The checklist for a good care atlas and the results of the expert interviews could serve as a guideline for planning and implementation.

The author agrees with the almost unanimous opinion of the experts that such a project should be started small in the sense of a quick win and further developed during operation. As the lowest common denominator for the go-live, he identifies a comprehensive presentation of all care services in the province of Salzburg. This lowest common denominator should be linked to the go-live by the forecast of population development and the biographical data of registered doctors, therapists, midwives and community nurses. The (data protection) legal, technical and (professional) political challenges arising from this appear to the author to be solvable.

As a first step towards implementation, he believes that a preliminary project group should be formed. Its central task should be to form a group of willing parties at regional level, whose commitment should be cast in legal form. Only then should the substantive work begin. Anything else would have meant putting the cart before the horse and would have led to "empty metres" and stranded costs. This could cause irreparable damage to the project and bring it down even before the actual start.

7.2 Limitations

The limitations result primarily from the requirements for this thesis: it is a Master's thesis. Both the author and his supervisor considered the number of eight expert interviews to be sufficient to achieve the necessary theoretical saturation (Merkens, 2009). The aim of qualitative research is not to test the reliability of precisely formulated hypotheses, but to describe reality, in this case the wishes and ideas of experts for a regional, cross-sectoral care atlas for the federal state of Salzburg, and thus help to make predictions (Kalle/Tempel, 2020). Further expert interviews, for example with IT specialists, care researchers, members of editorial teams of existing care atlases, representatives of the therapeutic professions, etc., would have been interesting, but were beyond the scope of this work.

The aim of this paper is to compile the basic content for a regional, cross-sectoral care atlas for the federal state of Salzburg. For this reason, it does not contain any estimates of the necessary personnel expenditure, possible costs or the time required for an implementation project. These points must be clarified when drawing up a project brief and the resulting project planning.

7.3 Conflicts of interest

The author is Head of Corporate Communications and Marketing at Salzburger Landeskliniken, a wholly owned subsidiary of the state of Salzburg. The realisation of a cross-sector care atlas for the province of Salzburg is a strategic project in the interests of the Salzburg provincial hospitals and their owner.

Bibliography

Augustin J, Kistemann T, Koller D, et al. Good Cartographic Practice in Health Care (GKPiG). Forum IfL, 32 ed: Leibnitz-Institut fur Landerkunde e. V. (IfL); 2017.

Augustin J, Scherer M, Augustin M, Schweikart J. [Health Atlases in Germany - An Overview]. Health Services. 2018;80(7):628-634.

Buhmann V, Fulop G, Lepuschutz L, Piso B. Health care. Regional differences. Atlases at a glance. Berlin: 17th German Congress for Health Services Research, 10-12 October 2018; 2018.

Federal Ministry of Social Affairs, Health, Care and Consumer Protection (2023). Austrian Health Structure Plan 2023.

Federal Ministry of Social Affairs, Health, Care and Consumer Protection/Gesundheit.gv.at (2024). Financing the public healthcare system. https://www.gesundheit.gv.at/gesundheitsleistungen/gesundheitswesen/finanzierung.html, accessed on 3 February 2024, 9.45 am.

Da-Cruz P, Herrmann T. Demographic change in hospitals: The neglected dimension: Deutsches Arzteblatt; 2010.

Degelsegger-Marquez A, Grubock A, Fidon IK. Health data in Austria - an overview. Vienna: Gesundheit Osterreich GmbH; 2022.

Development and Planning Institute for Health (EPIG). Regional Health Structure Plan - Salzburg 2025 - outpatient part. Presentation of outpatient care structures until 2025. Version 1.2 ed. Graz2019.

European Commission (2024). European Health Data Space (EHDS). https://health.ec.europa.eu/ehealth-digital- health-and-care/european-health-data-spacede, accessed 3. 2. 2024, 11.05 am.

Famira-Muhlberger U, Firgo M, Streicher G. Medical care and demographic change. Vol 8/2020: WIFO Monthly Reports; 2020.

Fletcher-Lartey S, Caprarelli G. Application of GIS technology in public health: successes and challenges. 143 ed: Parasitology; 2016. Furweger W. Demographic change in the province of Salzburg: effects on the healthcare system. Salzburg: Salzburg Provincial Hospitals; 2023.

Grote-Westrick M, Zich K, Klemperer D, et al. 2015: Bertelsmann Foundation; Faktenchek Gesundheit: Regionale Unterschiede in der Geundheitsversorgung im Zeitvergleich.

Hoffmann, W., Latza, U., Terschuren, C. Guidelines and recommendations for ensuring good epidemiological practice (GEP) - revised version after evaluation (2008). On the Internet: http://dgepi.de/ fileadmin/pdf/leitlinien/GEP_mit_Ergaezung_GPS_Stand_24.02.2009.pdf Status: 10.12.2014

Lubeck IfKeVldUz. Cancer Atlas for Schleswig-Holstein: https://www.krebsregister-sh.de, accessed on 19. 09. 2023, 16.07; 2023.
Kelle U, Tempel G. [Understanding through qualitative methods - the contribution of interpretative social research to health reporting]. Federal Health Gazette Health Research Health Protection. 2020;63(9):1126-1133.
Klemperer D, Robra B-P. Regional differences in care: John Wennberg - pioneer of patient-centred medicine. Vol 111(4): A-118/B-104/C-100: Deutsches Arzteblatt; 2014.
Koller D, Wohlrab D, Sedlmeir G, Augustin J. [Geographic methods for health monitoring]. Federal Health Gazette Health Research Health Protection. 2020;63(9):1108-1117.
Kuckartz U. Qualitative content analysis. Methods, practice, computer support (3rd edition). Weinheim/Basel: Beitz Verlag; 2016.
Province of Salzburg. Regional Health Structure Plan. Salzburg 2025. Acute inpatient part. 1.1 ed. Salzburg2019.
Mangiapane S. [Learning from regional differences: online platform: http://www.versorgungsatlas.de]. Federal Health Gazette Health Research Health Protection. 2014;57(2):215-223.
Mayring P. Qualitative content analysis. Basics and techniques (12th edition). Weinheim/Basel: Beitz Verlag; 2015.
McGlynn E, Asch S, Adams J, al. e. The quality of health care delivered to adults in the United States. Vol 348(26): New Enlgand Journal of Medicine; 2003.
Merkens H. Selection procedure, sampling, case construction. In: Flick, U.; von Kardorff, E.; Steinke, I. (eds.), Qualitative Forschung: ein Handbuch, 7th edition. ed. Reinbek: Rowohlt; 2009.
Meuser M, Nagel U. Expert interviews - often tested, little considered: a contribution to the qualitative methods discussion. In: Garz, Detlef/Kraimer, Klaus (eds.): Qualitativ-empirische Sozialforschung: Konzepte, Methoden, Analysen ed. Opladen: Westdeutscher Verlag; 1991.
Moen A, Goodman DC. Unwarranted geographic variation in paediatric health care in the United States and Norway. Acta Paediatr. 2022;111(4):733-740.
Mulley A, Trimble C, Elwyn G. Stop the silent misdiagnosis: patient's preferences matter: British Medical Journal; 2012.
NHS (2023). Atlas of Variation in Healthcare. https://finger-tips.phe.org.uk/profile/atlas-of-variation.
OECD. Tackling wasteful spending on health: https://www.oecd.org/health/tackling-wasteful-spending-on-health-9789264266414-en.htm, accessed 19. 09. 2023, 13.09.; 2017.

Paracelsus Medical University Salzburg (PMU, 2024). Centre for Public Health and Health Services Research. https://www.pmu.ac.at/zpv.html, accessed on 09.02.2024, 17.40.
Paris Lodron University Salzburg (PLUS, 2024). About IDA Lab. https://www.plus.ac.at/aihi/der-fachbereich/ida-lab/about/, accessed on 09/02/2024, 17:20.
Rammstedt B. Reliabilitat, Validitat, Objektivitat. In: Wolf, C., Best, H. (eds). Handbook of social science data analysis. ed. Wiesbaden: VS Verlag fur Sozialwissenschaften; 2010.
Austrian Court of Audit. Health data on pandemic management in the first year of the COVID-19 pandemic. Report of the Court of Audit. Vol Series BUND 2021/43, Series OBEROSTERREICH 2021/8; Series SALZBURG 2021/52021.
Robra BP. [John E. Wennberg, pioneer of regional health services research: what does he teach us in Germany?] Bundesgesund- heitsblatt Gesundheitsforschung Gesundheitsschutz. 2014;57(2):164-168.
Schang L, Morton A, DaSilva P, Bevan G. From data to decisions? xploring how healthcare payers respond to the NHS Atlas of Variation in Healthcare in England. Volume 114, Issue 1 ed: Health Policy; 2014.
Smith R. Dartmouth Atlas of Health Care. 2011;342:d1756 ed: BMJ. Spectrum of Science. Atlas of Geography. https://www.spek- trum.de, accessed 19. 09. 2023, 16.12.
Stacey D, Legare F, al. e. Decision aids for people facing health treatment or screening desicions. Vol 1: Cochrane Review; 2014.
Starke D, Tempel G, Butler J, Starker A, Zuhlke C, Borrmann B. Good Practice Health Monitoring - Guidelines and Recommendations 2.0. Vol 2019/4(S1): Journal of Health Monitoring; 2019.
Statistics Austria. Population forecast 2019, main variant. Vienna2019.
Statistics Austria (2024). Health expenditure. https://www.statistik.at/statistiken/bevoelkerung-und-soziales/gesundheit/gesundheitsversorgung-und-ausgaben/gesundheitsausgaben, accessed on 3 February 2024, 10.50 am.
Swart, E., Gothe, H., Geyer, S. et al. Good Practice Secondary Data Analysis (GPS): Guidelines and Recommendations. 3rd version; Version 2012, 2014, Public Health 2015; 77: 120-126.
Thiften M, Niemann H, Varnaccia G, et al. [What potential do geographic information systems have for population-wide health monitoring in Germany? : Perspectives and challenges for the health monitoring of the Robert Koch Institute]. Federal Health Gazette Health Research Health Protection. 2017;60(12):1440-1452.

Ulrich LR, Schatz TR, Lappe V, et al [Primary and secondary data on dementia care as an example of regional health planning]. Bundes-gesundheitsblattGesundheitsforschungGesundheitsschutz . 2017;60(12):1372-1382.

Weiss Susanne et al. Healthcare professions in Austria. Vienna: Federal Ministry of Social Affairs, Health, Care and Consumer Protection; 2023.

Wennberg J, Gittelsohn. Small area variations in health care delivery. Science. 1973;182(4117):1102-1108. doi: 1110.1126/science.1182.4117.1102.

Wennberg J. Tracking Medicine - A Researchers Quest to Understand Health Care. Oxford: University Press; 2010.

World Wide Web Consortium (W3G). Web Content Accessibility Guidelines (WCAG).

Central Institute for Statutory Health Insurance Physician Care (Zi). Supply atlas: https://www.versorgungsatlas.de/, accessed on 19. 09. 2023, 16.30; 2023.

Appendix

10.1 List of interview partners and their affiliations

- **Interview 1, Hospital:** Priv.-Doz. Dr Paul Sungler, Managing Director of Salzburger Landeskliniken from 2014 to 2023.
- **Interview 2, Administration:** Christian Prucher, Head of Department 9 (Hospitals and Healthcare) of the Salzburg Provincial Government.
- **Interview 3, social insurance:** Dr Peter Gruner, senior physician at the Salzburg regional office of the Austrian Health Insurance Fund.
- **Interview 4, panel doctor:** Dr Magdalena See- leitner, general practitioner with a panel practice in Salzburg- Aigen.
- **Interview 5, Nursing:** Magdalene Fischill-Neudeck MSc, Community Nurse in Thalgau.
- **Interview 6, Pharmacy:** Pharmacist Christina Sadlo, owner of the Gnigler pharmacy in the city of Salzburg.
- **Interview 7, patient representation:** Sabine Geistlinger, managing director of Selbsthilfe Salzburg (umbrella organisation of self-help groups).
- **Interview 8, Research:** Hofrat Dr Gernot Filipp MBA, Head of Department 0/24 (State Statistics and Administrative Controlling) of the Office of the Salzburg State Government

10.2 Interview guidelines

Interview guide

Phase 1: Explanation of the topic	***W*** Introduction of the interviewer in the context of the interview (Master's thesis and student and not speaker of the Salzburg state clinics). Explanation of the purpose of the survey. Presentation and delimitation of the topic.
Phase 2: Meaningfulness	***e*** How useful does a cross-sectoral atlas of healthcare provision in the province of Salzburg appear to be? ***e*** What purpose could or should a supply atlas fulfil for the province of Salzburg?
Phase 3: Scope	***e*** Should a Salzburg Health Atlas only serve health care research or also include epidemiological topics? ***e*** If it was also to include epidemiological topics: What were they and why?
Phase 4: Target groups	***e*** Which target groups should a cross-sectoral atlas of healthcare address? ***e*** Which groups of people or organisations should it not address?
Phase 5: Form of implementation	***g*** Should such an atlas be designed as a written report or digitally or digitally and interactively? ***e*** Should the development take place step by step - with a basis at the start and further modules in subsequent steps?
Phase 6: Contents for Start (Must-haves)	***n*** What content or functionalities should such an atlas definitely offer at go-live?
Phase 7: Possible further content (nice-to-haves)	Which content or functionalities should or could be implemented in the course of further steps. ***e*** Which content or functionalities should or could be implemented in the course of further steps.
Phase 8: Exclusion criteria (no-goes)	***e*** What content or functionalities can such an atlas not offer, or perhaps should it not offer at all?
Phase 9: Stumbling blocks	What major hurdles or challenges could arise during implementation?

Table 11: *Guidelines for the interviews with the selected experts.*

10.3 Criteria for a good supply atlas

Criteria for a good supply atlas	
Impartiality and acceptance	✓ The sponsor of the atlas is a public corporation, university, research institution or an association supported by public institutions. ✓ The sponsors are non-partisan and do not pursue any commercial interests with the atlas. ✓ The Atlas is subject to public control, e.g. by an advisory board or supervisory board, a parliamentary committee or a public control institution such as the Court of Auditors.
Scientificity	✓ Scientific claim - the purpose of the atlas is to gain knowledge and not, for example, to present political decisions. ✓ Spatial differences are described and discussed - new hypotheses can be generated from this. ✓ Reliability, validity and objectivity (intersubjectivity) (Wolf/Best, 2010) are ensured and formal criteria are adhered to in the presentation of maps and written reports. ✓ Guidelines such as Good Epidemiological Practice (Hoffmann et

	al., 2014), Good Practice in Secondary Data Analysis (Swart et al., 2015), Good Cartographic Practice in Healthcare (Augustin et al., 201 7) or Good Practice in Health Reporting (Starke et al., 2019) are adhered to.
Releva nce	✓ Quantity of data provided - high information content. ✓ The data is updated regularly. ✓ Benefits for the scientific community: The editorial team regularly publishes reports derived from the atlas and external authors can also publish articles on the atlas platform. ✓ (Local) external experts are involved in the interpretation of the results.
Accessibility and user-friendliness	✓ Clear and comprehensible visualisation of the data. ✓ Comprehensive and easy-to-understand introduction to usability and methodology. ✓ Interactive use is possible - e.g. zoom function, search and search filter, scroll function, customisation of the map legend, mouse-over function. ✓ Simple, intuitive handling - high usability. ✓ Extensive technical and textual accessibility. ✓ The data and reports are also available for printing or ✓ available for download. ✓ Users can submit comments and feedback and ask specific questions in accordance with the guidelines. ✓ Comprehensible summaries and interpretation aids are provided. ✓ Indications of limitations and possible interpretation errors.

Table 12: *Criteria for a good supply atlas - created by the author with input from Mangiapane (2014), Schang et al. (2014), Ulrich et al. (2017), Augustin et al. (2018), Koller et al. (2020).*

10.4 Results of the expert interviews in tabular form

Main category	Sub-category	Input from the experts
Category 1: Sense and purpose	Significance for society, the healthcare system and science	✓ Atlas provides new insights. ✓ Atlas unearths previously unused treasure trove of data. ✓ Atlas presents healthcare system without taboos. ✓ Atlas helps to ask questions and answer questions. ✓ Atlas supports networking in the healthcare system. ✓ Atlas is a guide for experts and health literate citizens. ✓ Atlas helps to manage patient flows. ✓ Atlas helps to keep people in the healthcare system in basic care for as long as possible and thus relieves the burden on outpatient clinics. ✓ Atlas contributes to the best possible outcome with the least possible effort.
	Objectives pursued	✓ Atlas provides stakeholders and the population with a low-threshold overview of supply structures. ✓ Atlas identifies supply shortages and under- or oversupply. ✓ Atlas takes into account the forecast population development. ✓ Atlas is the basis for forward-looking planning of supply structures and required resources.

		✓ Atlas contributes to the fair distribution of services among system partners. ✓ Atlas enables evaluation of decisions on supply structures. ✓ Atlas presents current and future necessary care structures for common diseases ("widespread diseases"). ✓ Atlas offers patients several options.
Category 2: Contents	Scope of the In ha lts	✓ Atlas depicts intramural and extramural structures down to municipal level. ✓ Atlas covers acute and long-term care as well as prevention and aftercare (rehabilitation facilities). ✓ Atlas shows which diseases are to be expected in which age groups. ✓ Atlas shows whether treatments are being carried out on time. ✓ Atlas is divided into sections for experts and laypersons (patients). ✓ Atlas also offers contact options for the recorded structures.
	Projects to be included	✓ Population forecast of the state statistics. ✓ Paracelsus 1 0,000" study. ✓ ELGA. ✓ SALK survey on demographic trends and hospitalisation rates.
Category 3: Target groups		✓ Key target groups are decision-makers from stakeholders in the healthcare system and patients. ✓ However, data is accessible to all interested persons (experts and laypersons).
Category 4: Form of realisation	Technology	✓ Atlas is a digital platform with cartographic representations that is as interactive as possible. ✓ Atlas differentiates between the target groups of stakeholders and patients. ✓ Reports and scientific contributions on individual topics complement the atlas. ✓ Results are available for downloading and printing.
	Organisation	✓ ***The sponsor is a public or scientific institution.*** ✓ ***Financing is provided by public funds.*** ✓ ***Atlas has fixed human and financial resources.*** ✓ ***Atlas starts with limited content and is then expanded.*** ✓ ***Fixes team is constantly gathering feedback, expanding, updating and maintaining Atlas.***
Category 5: Must-haves for the start	Law and organisation	✓ ***Clear will of the necessary stakeholders: Provincial politics, administration, hospitals, social insurance providers and professional organisations.*** ✓ ***Self-help groups, senior counselling services and representatives of inpatient and outpatient long-term care provide input.*** ✓ ***Atlas fulfils scientific requirements.*** ✓ ***Awareness of ethical responsibility - data can lead to the reorganisation or dismantling of structures.*** ✓ ***Valid data is also available for the future.*** ✓ ***Co-operation agreements also secure data flows for the future.***

	In ha lt or function	✓ ***Atlas provides an overview of all intramural and extramural structures down to municipal level.*** ✓ ***Atlas presents existing and future care structures for cardiovascular diseases, diabetes and brain health.*** ✓ ***Atlas provides contact details of the care structures.*** ✓ ***Feedback to the Atlas team is possible.*** ✓ ***Atlas displays the data geographically.*** ✓ ***Atlas offers a search function with filter options.*** ✓ ***Atlas offers download and print function.*** ✓ ***There are processes for ongoing updates.***
Category 6: Nice-to-haves in further operation	Contents	✓ ***Atlas visualises patient flows.*** ✓ ***Information brochures for patients are produced on the basis of the atlas.*** ✓ ***Atlas regularly provides up-to-date reports on specialised topics.*** ✓ ***Altas provides information on the functions and tasks of the healthcare professions.*** ✓ ***Atlas contains information on apprenticeships and vacancies.*** ✓ ***Atlas contains tips for self-help.*** ✓ ***Atlas presents complementary social offers.***
	Technology	✓ ***Atlas is available as an app for mobile devices.*** ✓ ***Atlas has advanced search and filter by symptoms.*** ✓ ***Atlas offers a ticket system for enquiries.*** ✓ ***Atlas offers scheduling coordination or jumping-off points for scheduling coordination.*** ✓ ***Reports are also available as podcasts.***
	Accompanying measures - little/no direct connection with the atlas.	✓ ***The atlas is widely advertised.*** ✓ ***There are terminals at public places as access points to the atlas.*** ✓ ***The establishment of medical group practices is being promoted.*** ✓ ***The non-medical extramural sector is being expanded.*** ✓ ***Pharmacies are increasingly integrated as part of the healthcare system.*** ✓ ***There are peers or guides through the healthcare system at local level.*** ✓ ***Prevention, health promotion and self-help are strengthened.*** ✓ ***The health literacy of the population is required.*** ✓ ***Financial flows in the healthcare system are simplified.*** ✓ ***The payment system is changed from the performance principle to the success principle.***
Category 7: No-Gos		✓ ***Atlas establishes links between clinical pictures and patients' ethnic origin, religion or sexual orientation.*** ✓ ***Atlas pursues economic interests.*** ✓ ***The pharmaceutical industry is a key partner of the Atlas.*** ✓ ***Churches and religious communities are integrated into the atlas.***
Category 8: Stumbling	Legal and systemic	✓ ***Changes in the healthcare system and demographics are not taken into account.***

blocks		✓ ***Too little consideration is given to data protection and data security.*** ✓ ***Ownership rights to the data are not taken into account.*** ✓ ***Lack of commitment from stakeholders/carriers - also for the future.*** ✓ ***Important stakeholders are not on board.*** ✓ Different (financial) interests of stakeholders. ✓ Suppliers of oversupply feel attacked. ✓ There is resistance from political parties and professional organisations. ✓ The population knows too little about the healthcare system, e.g. the GP system or the purpose of emergency departments.
	Project level	✓ The project is planned too large. ✓ The meaning and purpose of the project are communicated too little or unclear. ✓ Budget and personnel are not secured for the future. ✓ Key objectives and promises are not being fulfilled. ✓ Too much data leads to confusion. ✓ The focus - presentation of the data - is lost, technology becomes an end in itself.
	data	✓ Data is not up-to-date, incomplete or not robust. ✓ There are too many data sources. ✓ Data cannot be integrated due to missing interfaces. ✓ Data generation effort does not justify the result. ✓ Evaluation of data generation is missing. ✓ There is no standardised understanding of how to interpret the data. ✓ Data is transferred with incorrect interpretation - subsequent error. ✓ Processes for data generation and data transfer are not secured for the future. ✓ Data is not available for all participants.
	Target groups that cannot be reached or are not depicted	✓ The elective doctor sector is currently under-recorded. ✓ People from educationally disadvantaged backgrounds and with a migration background are difficult to reach. ✓ Many people, especially older people, have no or only poor internet access.

Table 13: *Results of the expert interviews in tabular form*

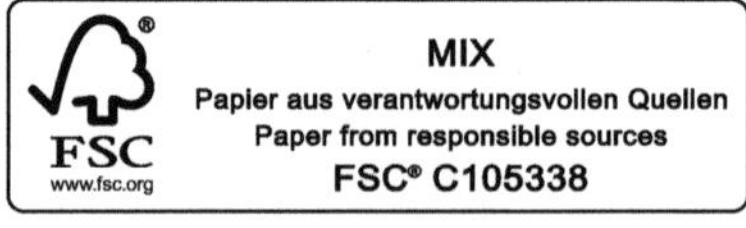

Printed by Books on Demand GmbH, Norderstedt / Germany